英汉消化系统疾病护理手册

English-Chinese Nursing Manual for Digestive Diseases

主审　李兆申　承　雨　郦　枫

主编　陈　翠　杜奕奇　陆小英

上海科学技术出版社

图书在版编目（ＣＩＰ）数据

英汉消化系统疾病护理手册 / 陈翠，杜奕奇，陆小英主编. -- 上海 ： 上海科学技术出版社，2024.6
ISBN 978-7-5478-6193-6

Ⅰ. ①英… Ⅱ. ①陈… ②杜… ③陆… Ⅲ. ①消化系统疾病－护理－手册－英、汉 Ⅳ. ①R473.57-62

中国国家版本馆CIP数据核字(2023)第086931号

英汉消化系统疾病护理手册

主审 李兆申 承 雨 郦 枫
主编 陈 翠 杜奕奇 陆小英

上海世纪出版(集团)有限公司
上 海 科 学 技 术 出 版 社 出版、发行
(上海市闵行区号景路159弄A座9F-10F)
邮政编码201101 www.sstp.cn
江阴金马印刷有限公司印刷
开本 889×1194 1/32 印张 4
字数 80千字
2024年6月第1版 2024年6月第1次印刷
ISBN 978-7-5478-6193-6/R·2771
定价：45.00元

内容提要

Synopsis

本书是为消化内科护理人员精心编撰的英汉双语手册，通过对各类消化内科护理临床情景的英文、中文描述和展示，帮助护理人员掌握基本的消化内科护理专业英语，以满足护理人员专业英语尤其是英语口语的学习需求和应用需求。本书共分三部分、38个专题，每个专题都列出了需要掌握、熟悉的护理内容及需要掌握的英文词汇，以查房对话的形式，从临床护理实际出发，对消化系统疾病患者的常规护理、消化疾病护理及专科导管护理等进行全面、深入浅出的阐释，方便消化内科护理人员在学习专业英语的同时，掌握消化内科护理知识和操作流程。

编者名单
Contributors

主　审

李兆申　承　雨　郦　枫

主　编

陈　翠　杜奕奇　陆小英

副 主 编

朱惠云　王　汇

编写秘书

印　坤

编　　者

（按姓氏汉语拼音排序）

陈　莉　柴计委　高　峻　李　芳　李　歌　梁金平

沈　慧　王春艳　杨盼瑞　印　坤　虞佳伟　张　艳

张　允　张红燕　赵大方　庄　璐　庄　颖　庄海花

序言一

Preface

消化系统结构特殊、功能复杂，疾病临床表现和诊疗手段多样。新理论、新技术的不断涌现和日趋频繁的国际交流，对消化内科专科护士提出了更高的要求。国家"十四五"规划纲要从战略高度强调了建设健康中国的重要意义，高水平的护理工作已成为提升医疗质量不可忽视的一部分。在发达国家，专科护士聚焦专业特色，蓬勃发展。在我国，专科护士培养近年来已成为护士职业发展的重要部分。

本书根据专科护士发展趋势，强调以整体护理为方向，以人的健康为中心，用简明的语言和临床工作中查房对话的形式，从临床护理实际出发，对消化系统疾病的一般知识、专科知识、导管知识等常规护理知识进行全面、深入浅出的阐释。本书编者中不仅有医学专家，还有国家消化系统疾病临床医学研究中心的护理团队。她们从消化系统疾病患者住院期间的需求出发，参考国内外文献，总结自身的专业知识和护理实践经验编写了本书，希望对护士日常护理工作有所裨益。

本书的出版，可提高护理人员对消化疾病的认识，也便于国际交流中让国际同仁更深入地了解我们的护理文化，对推动消化专科护理的发展有积极的作用。

李兆申

2023 年 11 月

序言二

Preface

消化内科学是一个具有特殊性的医学领域，消化系统涵盖了食管、胃、小肠、大肠、肝脏、胆囊和胰腺等多个器官，其所涉及的病种具有多样性和复杂性。另外，近年来随着科学技术的进步，消化内镜领域迎来了日新月异的发展。许多以前必须通过手术或介入手段才能进行诊治的疾病，现在通过先进的消化内镜技术便可得到及时而精准的诊断及治疗。该技术在安全性、舒适性、微创性和经济性诸多方面为患者和社会带来了前所未有的福音。消化内科学与外科学、放射学相辅相成，消化内镜技术的创新与进步推动了外科学及放射学的拓展。三个学科之间紧密的合作模式成功地为患者带来了最佳的治疗效果。

消化系统疾病的多样性、复杂性，以及消化内镜技术的前沿性和快速更新，也为消化内科的护理工作带来了挑战。在这方面我们与西方发达国家之间还存在着一定的差距。随着改革开放的进一步深入，国际交流的进一步深化，"一带一路"倡议的逐步实施，人类命运共同体已渐渐孕育成长。我国亟须大批优秀的消化内科护理人员借助流利、专业的英文来进行学习、教学、交流和工作，从而更好地为患者、为社会以及为世界服务。我们真诚地希望此书能在这一领域做一个探索者，发挥抛砖引玉的作用。

　　我在 18 岁时离开祖国到美国留学。当时英文基础几乎为零，而一年后进入了麻省理工学院进行本科学习。英文的学习及应用并非像很多人想象的那样难和可怕，只要心中有对医疗工作的热情和对患者的大爱，相信读者朋友们会找到适合自己的学习方法，并运用自己的智慧，克服学习中遇到的种种困难。最后，祝大家在生活和工作中不断发现和创造美，通过爱这把钥匙，开启幸福、成功之门。

郦枫

2023 年 11 月
于得克萨斯州

目 录

Contents

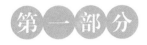

常规护理

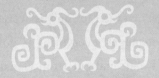

Part One

Routine Nursing

第一章 患者入院

Chapter 1 Patient check-in

1. 了解入院程序
2. 掌握下列词汇

nursing station 护士站
department of gastroenterology
　消化内科
inpatient ID card 住院证
diagnose 诊断（v.）
diagnosis 诊断（n.）

chronic pancreatitis 慢性胰
　腺炎
pressure ulcer 压疮
sacrococcygeal region 尾骶部
pay close attention to 对……
　加强关注

Li Ming comes to the nursing station of the Department of Gastroenterology. Liu Mei is on duty. On receiving the patient's inpatient ID card, Liu measures his height and weight, inputs data into the computer, and shows him around the ward.

Nurse manager: Hi Liu Mei, how is everything going?

Liu Mei: Hi manager, everything is going well. There is a new 65-year-old male patient from Gansu Province. He is diagnosed with chronic pancreatitis, and looks very thin. His BMI is below 18 kg/m^2, and he has severe stomachache. The pain grade is 6 out of 10. I have reported it to the doctor.

Nurse manager: Well done, Liu Mei. How about the patient's skin condition? Is there any pressure ulcer?

Liu Mei: There is no pressure ulcer. I have checked his sacrococcygeal region, back, and feet.

Nurse manager: Great job! In the next few days, please pay close attention to his skin, as the patient may not be able to turn over easily because of pain.

李明来到消化内科病房护士站，刘梅值班。她接到李明的住院证后，为李明测量身高和体重，数据录入电脑，并带他参观病房。

护士长：刘梅，患者情况怎么样？

刘梅：护士长好，一切都好，来了一位来自甘肃省诊断为慢性胰腺炎的65岁男性患者。患者看上去消瘦，BMI指数小于18 kg/m²，现在有严重的腹痛，疼痛评分6分，我已经向医生汇报。

护士长：做得不错，刘梅。这位患者皮肤怎样？有压疮问题吗？

刘梅：还没有，我已经检查了他的尾骶部、后背和足部。

护士长：很好！接下来的时间里，要重点关注患者的皮肤，因为疼痛导致他不能频繁地翻身。

第二章　安全宣教

Chapter 2　Patient safety education

 •••

1. 了解安全宣教内容
2. 掌握下列词汇

fast　禁食（v.）　　　　　　non-slippery slippers　防滑拖鞋

gastric tube　胃管　　　　　　pull up　拉起

Li Bo is a new patient aged over 80. Now he is fasting, and the doctor has placed a gastric tube into his stomach. His body skin is not damaged. Liu Mei, his primary nurse, is giving him safety instructions.

Liu Mei: Hello, Li Bo. I am Liu Mei, your primary nurse. Very nice to meet you. How are you feeling now?

Li Bo: I feel good. Thank you.

Liu Mei: You are at high risk of fall due to your age. Please prepare a pair of non-slippery slippers. Before sleep, you need to pull up the bed rails on both sides. You also need the company of your family 24 hours a day. To supplement more nutrition, the doctor has put a gastric tube in your body. Be careful not to pull it out when you move. You may do moderate bedside exercises and turn from side to side while lying in bed so as to prevent pressure ulcers. If you have any question, press the button any time. Here is the bedside bell.

Li Bo: Thank you very much.

李博是一位80多岁的新患者。他正在禁食，医生给他放置了一根胃管。他身上的皮肤没有破损。刘梅是他的责任护士，正在给他做安全宣教。

刘梅：你好，李博，我是你的责任护士刘梅，很高兴见到你。现在感觉怎样？

李博：我很好，谢谢。

刘梅：你年龄较大，属于跌倒高危人群。你需要准备一双防滑拖鞋，睡觉前要把两侧床栏拉起。你还需要24小时有家属陪伴。为了给你补充营养，医生给你留置了一根胃管。活动的时候小心一点，不要将胃管拔出。你可以在床旁适当活动，躺在床上的时候要左右翻身，防止发生压疮。如果你有任何问题，随时打铃呼叫我们，床头铃给你放在这里。

李博：非常感谢你！

第三章 患者评估

Chapter 3 Patient assessment

1.熟悉患者评估内容
2.掌握下列词汇

| collect of specimens 采集标本 | thermometer 体温表 |
| blood pressure and pulse (BP & P) 血压和脉搏 | draw one's blood 抽血 |

Su Fei is a newly admitted patient in bed #2. Liu Mei is her primary nurse. Liu Mei has completed the hospitalization education and accompanies Su Fei to the ward. She is now measuring the patient's vital signs and teaching her how to collect specimens.

Liu Mei: Hello, Su Fei, do you have any discomfort right now?

Su Fei: No, I am fine. Thank you.

Liu Mei: Please lie down. I am going to take your blood pressure and pulse. Do you have a history of high blood pressure?

Su Fei: No.

Liu Mei: OK, your blood pressure and pulse are normal. Here is the thermometer. Put it under your armpit, and keep it close to your skin for 5 minutes. (5 minutes later) Your temperature is also normal.

Su Fei: Thank you.

Liu Mei: We will draw your blood tomorrow morning. You

need to avoid food after 8 pm and avoid drink after 10 pm. You also need to collect stool and urine samples tomorrow morning, and collect your morning urine as your urine sample. Here are the specimen boxes.

Su Fei: Thank you very much.

Liu Mei: You're welcome. If you have any question, please call me any time.

苏菲是 2 床刚入院的患者，刘梅是她的责任护士。刘梅已经完成了入院宣教并送患者进入病房，现在正在给她测量生命体征并教她如何采集标本。

刘梅：你好，苏菲，现在有什么不舒服吗?

苏菲：谢谢，我很好。

刘梅：你先躺下来，我现在要给你测量血压和脉搏，请问你有高血压病史吗?

苏菲：没有。

刘梅：好的，你的血压和脉搏是正常的。这是体温表，放在你的腋下，紧贴着你的皮肤 5 分钟。（5 分钟后）你的体温也是正常的。

苏菲：谢谢。

刘梅：明天早上我们将会给你抽血，你需要今天晚上 8 点之后禁食，10 点之后禁水。你明天早上还需要留取大便和小便标本，小便标本留取晨尿，这些是标本盒。

苏菲：非常感谢。

刘梅：不用谢，有什么问题随时呼叫我。

第四章　医学检查

Chapter 4　Medical tests

 学习目标

1. 了解常规检查
2. 掌握下列词汇

> routine test　常规检查
> chest X-ray　X线胸片
> electrocardiogram (ECG)　心电图
> B-ultrasonography　B超
> checklist　检查单

Li Ming, a patient in bed #4, was admitted yesterday. He needs to do some routine tests today, including B-ultrasonography, electrocardiogram (ECG), and chest X-ray. Liu Mei is the duty nurse today. She is holding the checklist and instructing Li Ming about the tests.

Liu Mei: Good morning, Li Ming. How was your sleep last night?

Li Ming: Good morning. I had a very good sleep last night. Thank you.

Liu Mei: We need to do some tests for you today, including electrocardiogram (ECG), chest X-ray, and ultrasound exam. ECG examination is done in the ward. Chest X-ray examination is on the first floor of Building No.10, and ultrasonography examination is on the fourth floor of Building No.5. Are you still fasting this morning?

Li Ming: Yes, the nurse informed me last night.

Liu Mei: That's good. The abdominal B-ultrasonography requires an empty stomach. Please wait a moment. The medical assistant staff will pick you up for the exam.

Li Ming: OK, thank you.

 译文

　　4床患者李明是昨天入院的，他今天需要做一些常规检查，包括B超、心电图、X线胸片。护士刘梅今天值班，她正拿着检查单向李明宣教如何做这些检查。

　　刘梅：早上好，李明，昨天晚上睡得好吗？

　　李明：早上好，昨晚睡得很好，谢谢。

　　刘梅：今天需要做一些检查，包括心电图、X线胸片和B超。心电图检查是在病房做，X线胸片检查地点在10号楼一楼，B超检查地点在5号楼四楼。你早上还在禁食吗？

　　李明：是的，昨天晚上护士通知我了。

　　刘梅：那就好，你做的是腹部B超，需要禁食。请你稍等，护工会护送你去检查。

　　李明：好的，谢谢。

第五章 肠道准备

Chapter 5 Bowel preparation

1. 了解肠道准备的目的
2. 了解肠道准备常用药的机制
3. 掌握肠道准备的方法和注意事项
4. 掌握下列词汇

   constipation 便秘
   colonoscopy 肠镜
   bowel preparation 肠道准备
   polyethylene glycol (PEG) electrolyte power 聚乙二醇电解质散

Wang Gang has a constipation history and comes to the hospital for a comprehensive health checkup. He will have a colonoscopy tomorrow morning. Liu Mei, his primary nurse, is talking to him and giving him instructions regarding the bowel preparation before colonoscopy.

Liu Mei: Good morning, Wang Gang. The doctor will perform colonoscopy for you tomorrow morning. You need to clean out your bowels before the exam. Now I will tell you what to do.

Wang Gang: Ok, I am all ears.

Liu Mei: To improve the cleanliness of bowels, please have a low fiber half-liquid diet for lunch and dinner today, such as porridge, steamed bun, noodles, etc.

Wang Gang: OK!

Liu Mei: According to the doctor's advice, I will give you three bags of oral intestinal cleaner named polyethylene glycol (PEG) electrolyte powder, which is a volumetric laxative and will not cause water and electrolyte disturbance. Drink 1,000 mL warm water for each bag, which means 3,000 mL warm water for 3 bags. Drink 1,000 mL at 8 o'clock this evening and 2,000 mL at 5 o'clock tomorrow morning. It is recommended to drink 250 mL every 10 minutes and finish the drinking within 2 hours. It is common to experience abdominal discomfort during the process. If you have severe abdominal bloating or pain, you can slow down or stop it for a short period. You can resume taking it after the symptoms are gone. The goal is to leave no fecal residue in your body. Is everything clear?

Wang Gang: Yes, I think so.

Liu Mei: If you need more help, I'm always on call and ready to help you with the bowel preparation and check the defecation.

Wang Gang: Great, thank you so much, Liu Mei. I will keep your instructions in mind.

王刚有便秘病史，来医院做全面的医学检查。明天上午他要进行肠镜检查。刘梅是他的责任护士，正在和王刚谈话，告诉他肠镜前肠道准备的方法和注意事项。

刘梅： 早上好，王刚，明天上午医生将给你做肠镜检查，检查前需要清洁肠道，下面我将告诉你如何去做。

王刚：好的，我会认真听。

刘梅：为提高肠道清洁度，今天中饭和晚饭以低纤维半流质饮食为主，如粥、馒头、面条等。

王刚：好的。

刘梅：根据医生开具的医嘱，给你 3 袋口服肠道清洁剂，名称是聚乙二醇电解质散，它是容积性泻药，不会导致水和电解质紊乱，每袋用 1 000 mL 温开水冲服，3 袋共溶入 3 000 mL 温水，今天晚上 8 点喝 1 000 mL，明天早上 5 点喝 2 000 mL。建议每 10 分钟喝 250 mL，2 小时内喝完。在这个过程中腹部有不适是正常的，如有严重腹胀或不适，可放慢服用速度或暂停服用，待症状消除后再继续服用，腹泻直至体内没有粪渣。听明白了吗？

王刚：我基本清楚了。

刘梅：如果你需要，我可以帮你溶药和观察排便的情况。

王刚：好的，非常感谢你，刘梅，我会记住你的嘱咐。

第六章　介入术前宣教

Chapter 6　Pre-procedural education

 学习目标

1. 掌握介入术前的注意事项
2. 了解禁食、禁水的时间要求
3. 掌握皮试观察
4. 掌握下列词汇

polyp　息肉	induration　硬结
gastroscopy　胃镜	allergy test　过敏试验
skin test　皮试	

Wang Gang is a patient in bed #10. He is diagnosed with gastric polyps. Tomorrow he will get his polyps dissected by endoscopic polypectomy. Liu Mei, his primary nurse, is informing Wang Gang of important points before the procedure.

Liu Mei: Good morning, Wang Gang. The doctor will remove your polyps during gastroscopy tomorrow. I'm here to give you some instructions.

Wang Gang: Ok, I will listen carefully.

Liu Mei: You should fast for at least 8 hours before the operation. Avoid drinking for 2 hours or more. Take an anti-foam simethicone orally to facilitate mucosal inspection 30 minutes before endoscopy.

Wang Gang: Ok!

Liu Mei: According to the doctor's advice, cephalosporin will be administered to treat infection. And we need to do cephalothin allergy test now. Have you ever taken cephalosporin before? Do you have a history of food allergies and allergic diseases? Do your family members have the history of food allergy or severe allergy to medicine?

Wang Gang: Not as far as I know.

Liu Mei: The cephalosporin intradermal skin test is finished, and I will come to check the result after 20 minutes. During this period, in case of any discomfort, such as chest tightness, itching, facial numbness and fever, call me immediately. We will keep a close eye on you.

Twenty minutes later.

Liu Mei: Wang Gang, time is up. Let me have a look at the skin test site. Um, there is no redness or other change in the test site. Do you have any other discomfort?

Wang Gang: No, I am feeling good.

Liu Mei: Well, your skin test turns out negative. Thank you for your cooperation!

Wang Gang: Good, thanks a lot. I will keep your instructions in mind.

王刚是 10 床患者，他被诊断为胃息肉，明天他要行胃镜下息肉摘除手术。刘梅是王刚的责任护士，正在和他谈话，告

诉他介入术前重要的注意事项。

刘梅：早上好，王刚，医生安排你明天做胃镜下息肉摘除术，现在我来告诉你注意事项。

王刚：好的，我会认真听。

刘梅：术前你需要禁食至少 8 小时、禁水至少 2 小时，术前 30 分钟口服祛泡剂和祛黏液。

王刚：好的。

刘梅：根据医生开具的医嘱，术后治疗感染，一般会使用头孢菌素类抗生素。现在需做头孢菌素过敏试验，请问你使用过头孢类菌素类抗生素吗？有食物过敏史及过敏性疾病史吗？你的家人有食物或药物过敏史吗？

王刚：据我所知都没有。

刘梅：现在我给你做好了头孢菌素皮试，20 分钟后我来看检查结果。在这期间如果有胸闷、瘙痒、面部发麻、发热等不适，请你立即呼叫我，我也会多来看望你的。

20 分钟后。

刘梅：王刚，时间到了，让我来看看皮试结果，嗯，没有红晕，范围也没有变化，你有其他不舒适的吗？

王刚：不，我感觉还好。

刘梅：好的，你的皮试结果是阴性的，谢谢你的配合。

王刚：好的，非常感谢你，我会记住你的嘱咐。

第七章 介入术后宣教

Chapter 7 Post-procedural education

1. 了解介入术后输液的作用
2. 了解低血糖的症状
3. 掌握下列词汇

   intervention procedures　介入　　　intravenous fluids　静脉输液
   　　治疗　　　　　　　　　　　　　hypoglycemia　低血糖症

Wang Gang has undergone endoscopic polypectomy and just returned to the ward. Liu Mei is his primary nurse. She is telling him about what to do after interventional procedures.

Liu Mei: Hi, Wang Gang. How are you feeling now?

Wang Gang: Quite good, but I feel a bit hungry and weak.

Liu Mei: Don't worry. It is very common to feel like this, as you have been fasting for more than 8 hours. I will give you some intravenous fluids according to the doctor's instructions.

Wang Gang: That would be great. Thank you!

Liu Mei: My pleasure. Now I am giving you an intravenous infusion of 5% glucose. If you still have symptoms, such as dizziness, cold sweat, palpitation, hunger, and trembling, that means you have hypoglycemia. Just call me immediately and I will come right away.

Wang Gang: Ok, I feel much better now. Thank you, Liu Mei.

Liu Mei: You're welcome. Have a good rest.

王刚完成了胃镜下息肉摘除介入治疗，刚刚回到病房。刘梅是王刚的责任护士，正在和他谈话，告诉他介入术后重要的注意事项。

刘梅： 你好，王刚，现在感觉怎么样？

王刚： 我挺好的，就是感觉有点饿，没有力气。

刘梅： 很多患者在术后都会有这种饥饿感，因为超过 8 小时没有进食了，你不要太紧张，根据医生的医嘱，我马上给你静脉输液。

王刚： 那太好了，谢谢你！

刘梅： 不客气，现在我给你输液，输注的液体是 5% 葡萄糖，如果你还有头晕、出冷汗、心慌、饥饿、颤抖等症状，说明你出现了低血糖，请立即呼叫我，我会马上过来看你的。

王刚： 好的，我现在感觉好多了，谢谢你，刘梅！

刘梅： 不客气，你好好休息吧！

第八章　心理护理

Chapter 8　Mental health nursing

 学习目标

1. 掌握肿瘤患者的心理护理
2. 掌握下列词汇

therapy	治疗方法	upset	心烦意乱的
radiotherapy	放射疗法	diet	饮食
chemotherapy	化学疗法	hematemesis	呕血

Zhang Jun is a patient diagnosed with gastric cancer. He comes to the hospital for treatment. Li Na is his primary nurse. She is talking with Zhang Jun and giving him an education.

Li Na: Good morning, Zhang Jun. How do you feel today?

Zhang Jun: Good morning, Li Na. I am quite worried about my illness and scared of death.

Li Na: I fully understand your feeling, Zhang Jun. Having cancer does not mean you are going to die. There are many therapies available now, such as radiotherapy, chemotherapy and so on.

Zhang Jun: I do not know whether they work for me or not, which makes me even more upset.

Li Na: I do understand. Actually, mental state and emotions would have a direct impact on the treatment outcome. So a positive state of mind can help you achieve the best outcome.

Zhang Jun: OK, I will try to stay positive. What about my diet?

Li Na: Please eat small but frequent meals, say, five to six meals per day. Adjust the amount of food for each meal according to your comfort level. Eat slowly and chew the food fully so as to mix it well with the saliva, which works just like the stomach.

Zhang Jun: Well, I've written them down. What should I do after I return home?

Li Na: You need to keep a regular way of life, avoid getting fatigued and keep a positive mental state. Come back for regular checkups. Seek medical attention immediately once you have stomachache, hematemesis or black stool. Stop smoking or drinking alcohol, and avoid catching a cold.

Zhang Jun: OK, thank you, Li Na.

张军患有胃癌，到医院进行治疗，李娜是他的责任护士，正在和张军对话，进行健康教育。

李娜：早安，张军，今天感觉怎么样？

张军：早安，李娜，我很担心自己的疾病，我害怕死亡。

李娜：我理解你的感受，张军，身患癌症并不等于死亡，现在很多方法进行治疗，比如放射治疗、化学治疗等。

张军：不知道疗效怎么样，这让我很担心。

李娜：我理解你的心情。其实态度和情绪会直接影响治疗效果，所以你要保持积极乐观的心态，才能达到最理想的治疗效果。

张军：好吧，我尽量保持积极乐观的心态。在饮食上有什么注意的？

李娜：饮食上要少食多餐，每日 5～6 次，食量以自我感觉无不适为宜，进食一定要细嚼慢咽，使食物在口腔内充分嚼烂，与唾液充分混合，就像胃的运动。

张军：哦，我记下来了，回家之后要注意什么呢？

李娜：生活要有规律，避免劳累，保持乐观的心态。定期复查，有胃痛、呕血、黑便及时就诊。戒烟、戒酒，避免感冒。

张军：好的，谢谢你，李娜。

第九章　疼痛护理
Chapter 9　Pain management

 学习目标

1. 了解疼痛的药物指导
2. 掌握下列词汇

chronic pain　慢性疼痛　　　　　dosage　剂量，用量

oral administration　口服给药

Zhang Jun suffers from chronic pain and comes to the hospital for pain control. Li Na is his primary nurse. She is talking with the patient and giving health instructions.

Li Na: Good morning, Zhang Jun. How do you feel today?

Zhang Jun: Good morning, Li Na. I am sorry to tell you that I didn't take the medication last night as I had no pain. Now I'm feeling quite painful.

Li Na: Sorry to hear that. We regularly dispense medications to you based on its half-life and duration. The purpose is to provide continuous pain relief. If you do not take the medicine on time, it would be difficult to keep your pain under control.

Zhang Jun: Why do I need to take oral pain relievers?

Li Na: Oral administration of medicine is more economical, convenient and provides better absorption and greater safety.

Zhang Jun: Okay, Li Na. I will take medicine on time, but I am wondering why other people take less dose of pain medicine than I do.

Li Na: Good question. Because the sensitivity to narcotic drugs varies greatly among individuals, there is no universal dosage of opiates for all people. The optimal dosage is the one that can relieve pain and minimize side effects.

Zhang Jun: OK, I understand. But the pain really bothers me.

Li Na: Don't worry. Your pain can be relieved. Do not endure the pain when it occurs. Instead, you should tell us your pain score immediately so that we can make the right management plan for you. Take oral drugs on time. Do not stop drugs or alter the dosage and the frequency of drug-taking without physician's advice.

Zhang Jun: OK. Thank you, Li Na. This conversation makes me feel much better.

张军患有慢性疼痛，他来医院控制疼痛。李娜是他的责任护士，她正在和患者对话，进行健康教育。

李娜： 早安，张军，今天感觉怎么样？

张军： 早安，李娜，对不起，昨天晚上没有痛，所以药物没有按时吃，今天感觉肚子很痛。

李娜： 听到这些我很遗憾，我们是按照药物的半衰期及作用时间，定时给你发药，目的是使疼痛得到持续的缓解。如果你没有按时吃药，那么你的疼痛会很难控制。

张军： 为什么一定要口服止痛药呢？

李娜：口服给药经济、方便、吸收好、安全性高。

张军：好吧，李娜，我一定按时吃药，但是很奇怪，为什么别人吃的药量比我少？

李娜：这个问题问得好。因为麻醉药品的敏感度个体差异很大，所以阿片类药品并没有标准剂量，凡是能使疼痛得到缓解并且不良反应最低的剂量就是最佳剂量。

张军：好的，我记住了，但是疼痛真的让我很苦恼。

李娜：不要太担心，疼痛是可以缓解的。不要忍痛，疼痛发生时，及时告知我们疼痛评分，以便我们可以制订正确的镇痛方案。口服药物要按时服用，不可擅自停药或增减药量及频次。

张军：好的，谢谢你李娜，这次交谈让我安心很多。

第十章 肿瘤化疗护理

Chapter 10 Tumor chemotherapy nursing

 学习目标

1. 了解化疗饮食指导
2. 了解化疗常见不良反应
3. 掌握下列词汇

chemotherapy 化疗	nausea 恶心
side effect 副作用	vomit 呕吐
metabolic 新陈代谢的	antiemetic drug 止吐药
leukopenia 白细胞减少症	

Zhang Jun is a patient in bed #15 who has been diagnosed with malignant tumors. He comes to the hospital for chemotherapy. Li Na is his primary nurse. She is talking with the patient and giving him a health instruction.

Li Na: Good morning, Zhang Jun. How was your sleep last night?

Zhang Jun: Good morning, Li Na. I had a good sleep.

Li Na: You will undergo an intravenous chemotherapy this time.

Zhang Jun: Well, I am a bit worried. How about my diet during this procedure?

Li Na: You need to eat a variety of foods before chemotherapy. The foods should be low in fat, high in protein and vitamin and easy to digest. Besides three meals a day, you may also have tea breaks and night snacks. One day before chemotherapy, you should reduce the intake of sugar and grease, and eat fresh fruits and vegetables which are rich in vitamins. During the 24 hours after chemotherapy, you are advised to eat light meal, as taste may change due to the side effects of chemotherapy. A moderate amount of lean meat, fruits and vegetables, beans, and egg white is also recommended. Your body functions cannot return to normal shortly after chemotherapy. During this period, you should choose easy-to-digest food, and eat small but frequent meals. Slow down when you drink and eat and avoid high-fat, fried, sweet, and greasy foods. Choose foods that are colorful and delicious enough to increase your appetite. You may also take a moderate amount of foods rich in vitamin C, such as fruits and vegetables, which help to prevent constipation, boost immune system, and facilitate the recovery. Drink plenty of water to promote metabolism. Stay away from perfume, cigarettes, and kitchen fumes.

Zhang Jun: Okay, thank you, Li Na. Could you tell me something about the side effects and precautions of chemotherapy?

Li Na: Because of the fundamental metabolic differences between cancer cells and normal cells, chemotherapeutic drugs can cause some damage to normal tissues and induce various reactions while killing cancer cells. For example, you might lose hair during and after the treatment. But in general, your hair will start to grow two to three months after the chemotherapy. Bone marrow suppression may also occur. Leukopenia will cause a decline in immunity. According to the blood test results, we may use medications to increase your white blood cell count when necessary. Reduction in platelet count might occur and lead to spontaneous and hard-to-stop bleeding. Therefore, you need to spend more time in bed and brush teeth with soft-hair toothbrush. Press the injection spot for five to ten minutes after extraction of the needle. Rinse your mouth after meal to prevent oral ulcers. Eat foods rich in coarse fiber. In case of nausea or vomiting, we are going to give you injection of antiemetic drugs.

Zhang Jun: OK, thank you, Li Na. I will keep your advice in mind.

　　张军是 15 床患者，他患有恶性肿瘤，到医院进行化疗。李娜是他的责任护士，她正在和患者对话，进行健康教育。

　　李娜： 早安，张军，昨天休息的怎么样？

　　张军： 早安，李娜，昨天休息的还可以。

　　李娜： 这次入院要进行静脉药物化疗。

　　张军： 是的，我有点紧张，用药期间饮食上需要注意什么？

　　李娜： 化疗前期食物应当做到多样化，选择低脂肪、高蛋白质、多维生素和易消化的食物，除了一日三餐，还可以适当增加下午茶和宵夜。接受化疗前一天，应减少糖分、油脂的摄入，多吃富含维生素的新鲜果蔬。在接受化疗的 24 小时内，饮食要清淡，因为在不良反应的影响下口味会发生变化。可以吃适量瘦肉、果蔬、豆类和蛋清。化疗结束后，身体功能短时间内无法恢复至正常状态，在此期间吃易消化的食物，少食多餐，喝水和吃饭速度不宜过快；勿食高脂、油炸、甜腻食物；食物要色香味俱全，以增进食欲。适当吃些富含维生素 C 的食物，如水果、蔬菜，起到防止便秘、提高免疫力的作用，有利于化疗后的恢复。多饮水，促进药物代谢。远离香水、香烟、油烟等气味。

张军：好的，谢谢你，李娜，你能不能给我说说化疗有哪些不良反应和注意事项？

李娜：由于肿瘤细胞和正常细胞之间存在根本性的代谢差异，化疗药物在杀死肿瘤细胞的同时也会对正常组织产生一定的损伤而引起不同的反应。比如，会出现脱发，但一般停用化疗药 2～3 个月会长出新发。比如，会出现骨髓抑制，白细胞减少会引起身体抵抗力下降，根据血化验结果，必要时使用升高白细胞的药物；血小板减少容易出血，要多卧床休息，用软毛牙刷刷牙，拔针后按压 5～10 分钟。餐后漱口，预防口腔溃疡。多吃粗纤维食物，预防便秘等。如果有恶心、呕吐，我们会给你注射止吐药物。

张军：好的，谢谢你，李娜，我会认真牢记你的建议。

第十一章 交班

Chapter 11　Shift change

 学习目标

1. 掌握交班汇报内容及流程
2. 掌握以下词汇

　hypertension　高血压病
　extracorporeal shock wave lithotripsy (ESWL)　体外冲击波碎石
　physical cooling　物理降温

Good morning everyone, I am the night-shift nurse. During the past 24 hours, 2 patients checked out, 2 patients checked in and 8 patients received interventional therapies. Right now there are 28 patients in the ward, with 12 under primary care.

Check-out patients:

Wang Ming, bed #3, diagnosed with chronic pancreatitis.

Chen Yang, bed #18, diagnosed with Crohn's disease.

They checked out yesterday.

Check-in patients:

Wang Gang, bed #3, diagnosed with chronic pancreatitis. He comes on foot and can take care of himself independently, over 10-year history of hypertension, blood pressure well controlled by regular medicine, no discomfort during the night.

Liu Xin, bed #18, diagnosed with acute pancreatitis. He comes with the help of others, with limited independence in life and history of penicillin allergy.

Patients receiving operations:

Wang Qi, bed #5, diagnosed with chronic pancreatitis; received extracorporeal shock wave lithotripsy (ESWL) yesterday; no bloating or abdominal pain after the procedure; good sleep last night.

Li Guang, bed #12, diagnosed with chronic pancreatitis; received ESWL yesterday; nausea after the procedure; further observation is suggested by the doctor.

Patients with changed conditions:

Chen-xi Wang, bed #2, diagnosed with pancreatic cancer; body temperature 38.2℃ 6 pm yesterday; using ice packs for physical cooling as directed by the doctor; body temperature 36.9℃ thirty minutes after the cooling; 36.2℃ 6 am today.

Patients to undergo ESWL today:

Liu Juxiang, bed #6, and Zhang Yu, bed #9.

Nothing special with other patients. Over.

大家早上好，我是夜班的责任护士。在过去 24 小时内，出院 2 人，入院 2 人，介入治疗患者 8 人。目前病房患者总数 28 人，其中一级护理 12 人。

出院患者：3 床患者王明，诊断为慢性胰腺炎；18 床患者陈洋，诊断为克罗恩病，这 2 位患者均于昨日出院。

入院患者： 3床患者王刚，诊断为慢性胰腺炎，患者步行入病房，生活无需依赖，既往有高血压病史10余年，规律服药，血压平稳，晚夜间无不适，睡眠好。

18床患者刘鑫，诊断为急性胰腺炎，患者被搀扶入病房，生活轻度依赖，青霉素过敏。

介入治疗的患者： 5床患者王旗，诊断为慢性胰腺炎，昨日行体外冲击波碎石术，术后无腹胀、腹痛，夜间睡眠好。

12床患者李光，诊断为慢性胰腺炎，昨日行体外冲击波碎石术，术后感觉恶心，医生建议加强观察。

一般病情交班： 2床患者王晨曦，诊断为胰腺癌，昨日18：00体温38.2℃，遵医嘱给予冰袋物理降温，30分钟后复测体温36.9℃，今晨6：00体温36.2℃。

今日手术名单： 6床患者刘菊香和9床患者张宇均行体外冲击波碎石术。

其余患者无特殊，交班完毕。

第十二章 患者出院

Chapter 12 Patient check-out

 学习目标

1. 掌握出院结账办理及饮食宣教
2. 掌握以下词汇

discharge certificate　出院证　　　greasy　油腻的，高脂的

Liu Mei: Hi, Xiao Zhan. You've been recovering quite well recently. According to the doctor's order, you can check out today.

Xiao Zhan: Really? That is great!

Liu Mei: You need to check out with the discharge certificate, discharge summary and deposit receipt.

Xiao Zhan: Thank you. Can I use mobile payment?

Liu Mei: Yes. Besides mobile payment, you can also pay with bank card or cash.

Xiao Zhan: Thank you. What should I do after discharge? Any suggestions?

Liu Mei: Eat more fresh vegetables and fruits. Avoid greasy, cold, and hard food. Do moderate and non-strenuous exercises, such as walking and Tai Ji.

Xiao Zhan: Thanks again for your advice.

Liu Mei: Please make sure you've taken everything with you.

Xiao Zhan: I think so. Thanks a lot.

Liu Mei: My pleasure. It's our duty. Do not stop medication and come back for regular checkups. See the doctor as soon as possible if your condition gets worse.

Xiao Zhan: Thank you very much.

刘梅：你好，肖战。近期恢复得不错，根据医生医嘱你可以出院了。

肖战：是真的吗？那太好了！

刘梅：拿着出院证、出院小结、押金单就可以办理出院了。

肖战：谢谢，我可以手机支付吗？

刘梅：你可以用手机、银行卡或者现金支付。

肖战：谢谢，出院后我应该注意什么？有什么建议？

刘梅：多吃新鲜蔬菜水果，忌吃油腻、生冷坚硬的食物，适当运动，以身体耐受为宜，例如散步、打太极。

肖战：再次感谢你的建议。

刘梅：请确认没有遗忘物品。

肖战：应该没有，非常感谢。

刘梅：不用谢！这是我们的职责。坚持吃药，定期到医院复查，一旦病情变化，马上看医生。

肖战：非常感谢！

第十三章 电话回访
Chapter 13 Telephone follow-up

 学习目标

1. 掌握电话回访内容
2. 掌握以下词汇

up-date 最新消息   dull pain 钝痛
belly 腹部   recovery 恢复，康复

Nurse: Hi, I am a nurse of gastroenterology department, Changhai Hospital. My name is Yang Jin.

Patient: Hello, this is Liu Jun speaking.

Nurse: Do you have a minute? I need to have an up-date of your physical condition?

Patient: Sure.

Nurse: How have you been these days?

Patient: Quite well, except for occasional discomfort and dull pain in my belly.

Nurse: Do you take medication regularly?

Patient: Yes, I am already tired of taking medicine every day.

Nurse: I know it is hard for you. But an old saying goes that good medicine tastes bitter. Have you seen the doctor again?

Patient: Yes, the doctor said that my recovery is going well.

There is no need to worry about it.

Nurse: OK, great.

Patient: Any suggestions about my diet?

Nurse: Of course. Eat more fresh fruits and vegetables; choose foods that are easy to digest; avoid fried, uncooked and cold foods; do moderate exercises and don't lie in bed immediately after meals.

Patient: Thank you. I will follow your advice.

Nurse: You're welcome. Stay in touch.

Patient: Thank you for your care. Goodbye.

Nurse: Goodbye.

译文

护士：你好，我是长海医院消化内科的护士杨锦。

患者：你好，我是刘军。

护士：我能否耽误你两分钟，了解一下你最近的身体状况？

患者：可以，你请讲。

护士：你现在身体怎么样？

患者：最近身体还可以，就是有时肚子不舒服，隐隐作痛。

护士：你有规律服药吗？

患者：是的，我已经害怕每天吃药了。

护士：我知道这不容易，俗话说良药苦口利于病，你去医院复查过吗？

患者：是的，医生说恢复得挺好，不用担心。

护士：好的。

患者：饮食方面可以给我一些建议吗？

护士：多吃一些新鲜蔬菜水果，易消化的食物，少吃油炸生冷的东西，饭后要适当运动，不要立即躺在床上。

患者：谢谢，我会听从你的建议。

护士：不客气，保持联系。

患者：谢谢你的关心，再见。

护士：再见。

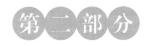

第二部分

消化疾病护理

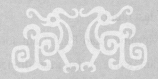

Part Two

Digestive Disease Care

第一章　胃食管反流病

Chapter 1　Gastroesophageal reflux disease

 学习目标

1. 了解疾病发生机制
2. 熟悉刺激胃酸分泌的食物
3. 掌握饮食指导、药物宣教
4. 掌握以下词汇

regular diet　规律饮食　　　　heartburn　胃灼热
stomachache　胃痛

Zhang Jun has severe symptoms of acid reflux, heartburn and bloating, and is clinically diagnosed with gastroesophageal reflux disease (GERD). He comes to the hospital for reflux control. His primary nurse Xiao Ran is talking with Zhang Jun and giving him a health instruction.

Xiao Ran: Morning, Zhang Jun. It's a sunny day today. Any unusual discomfort last night?

Zhang Jun: Morning Xiao Ran! I am sorry I did not follow your advice and drank some coffee after dinner, as I didn't finish my engineering drawings until 2 o'clock this morning, I am not feeling well right now, with noticeable stomachache, heartburn, and acid reflux.

Xiao Ran: Oh, I am sorry to hear that. You have so much

work to do, even in the hospital. If you cannot keep a regular diet and have enough rest, it is difficult to cure GERD.

Zhang Jun: Could you tell me again what foods I should avoid? I will take your suggestions seriously this time.

Xiao Ran: OK, Zhang Jun. First, you should try to maintain a regular lifestyle, including work, diet, and enough rest. You'd better eat easy-to-digest meals. Poached and steamed foods are better choices than fried foods. Caffeine, which is commonly found in coffee and strong tea, may cause heartburn. After meal you'd better sit for 30 minutes and do not lie down immediately. Especially after dinner, it is recommended to walk for an hour. Use a high pillow during sleep.

Zhang Jun: Thank you so much, Xiao Ran. I will bear your advice in mind.

　　张军有非常严重的反酸、烧心和腹胀症状，临床诊断为胃食管反流病。此次为控制胃酸反流入院，小冉是他的责任护士，她正在和患者对话并给予张军健康教育。

　　小冉：早安张军，今天天气晴好！昨晚有无特殊不适？

　　张军：早安小冉！抱歉，我没有遵循你的建议，晚饭后喝了咖啡。昨晚绘制工程图直到凌晨2点。现在我感觉不舒服，有明显的胃痛、胃灼热和胃酸反流。

　　小冉：哦，我很抱歉听到这些，你有很多工作要做，甚至在医院里都停不下来。如果你不能管理好饮食和休息时间，那么很难治愈胃食管反流病。

张军：你能不能告诉我什么食物不能吃？这次我会认真听从你的建议。

小冉：好的，张军。首先，你应该尽量保持规律的生活和休息，包括工作、饮食和充分的休息。我建议你吃易消化的食物，水煮和蒸食比油炸食品更适合你。浓茶、咖啡里含咖啡因，会引发胃部灼热感。吃完食物后，最好坐 30 分钟，不要立刻躺下。特别是在晚饭后，建议散步 1 个小时，睡觉时需要一个较高的枕头。

张军：非常感谢你小冉！我会牢记你的建议。

第二章　贲门失迟缓症

Chapter 2　Achalasia of cardia

1. 了解 POEM 围手术期护理
2. 掌握疾病指导与宣教
3. 掌握以下词汇

achalasia　失迟缓症   malnutrition　营养不良

dysphagia　吞咽困难   complication　并发症

nausea　恶心   esophagus　食管

vomit　呕吐   countermeasure　干预措施

Liu Xiang is a patient in bed #5. He suffers from severe achalasia, with constant dysphagia, nausea and vomiting, chest pain, recurrent lung infections, and moderate malnutrition. He comes to the hospital for treatment. Lin Yun is his primary nurse. She is talking with Liu Xiang and giving him a health instruction.

Lin Yun: Good afternoon, Liu Xiang. Tomorrow you will undergo the peroral endoscopic myotomy (POEM). Do you know what to do before the operation?

Liu Xiang: Good afternoon, Lin Yun. This is my first hospitalization. I hope you can tell me what I am supposed to do.

Lin Yun: Sure. First, relax yourself and have trust in us. Second, fast for 12 hours before the procedure. Finally, do not eat or drink anything after the operation until your doctor allows you to.

Liu Xiang: OK, will I have any discomfort after the operation?

Lin Yun: There may be some complications. But don't worry, since we have countermeasures. For example, you might get an infection after the operation, and we will give you antibiotics when it occurs.

Liu Xiang: OK, thank you. What am I supposed to do afterwards?

Lin Yun: Certainly, you need to wear baggy clothes to avoid abdominal pressure increase. In addition, while sleeping, raise the head of the bed by 10-15 cm to help empty the esophagus. As for diet, eat small but frequent meals, and choose soft and calorie-rich foods with plenty of nutrients.

Liu Xiang: OK, thank you very much. I will take your advice.

　　刘翔是 5 床患者，他有非常严重的贲门失迟缓症，常有吞咽困难、恶心、呕吐、胸痛的感觉，有反复的肺部感染，伴有中度营养不良。他来医院接受治疗，林允是他的责任护士，她正在与刘翔对话，并对他进行健康宣教。

　　林允： 中午好刘翔！明天你要做经内镜下环行肌切开手术（POEM），你知道手术前应该准备什么吗？

　　刘翔： 中午好林允！这是我第一次住院，我不太懂，希望你能教我！

　　林允： 好的。首先，你应该放松你的心情，不要太紧张，请相信我们的技术水平；其次，手术前大约 12 个小时你需要停止饮水，也就是说今晚 8 点以后你就不能饮水了；最后，手术结束后回到病房，你还是需要禁水，直到医生允许你饮水。

刘翔：好的，手术以后我会有不舒服症状吗？

林允：可能会有一些的，但是你不要紧张，我们有对症治疗措施！比如，术后可能会出现感染，我们会给你使用抗生素。

刘翔：好的，谢谢你们！那我以后需要注意什么吗？

林允：当然了，你以后要穿宽松的衣服，这样可以避免腹压增高；另外，睡觉的时候要把床头抬高 10～15 cm，这样可以促进食管排空。在饮食方面，要注意饮食习惯，尽量少量多餐，选择柔软而富含热量的食物，补充充足的营养。

刘翔：好的，非常感谢你！我一定会听从你的意见！

第三章 食管癌

Chapter 3　Esophageal cancer

1. 食管狭窄的治疗手段
2. 内镜下食管扩张术的优点
3. 掌握以下词汇

swallow　吞咽	dilatation　扩张
esophageal stenosis　食管狭窄	trauma　创伤
be scheduled to　计划安排	

Li Ming was diagnosed with esophageal cancer 3 years ago. Currently he has difficult eating and swallowing. He has been diagnosed with esophageal stenosis after the examination and is waiting for an operation tomorrow.

Nurse: Good morning Li Ming. How are you today?

Li Ming: Not too bad.

Nurse: Your operation is scheduled tomorrow. Has your doctor told you about it?

Li Ming: Yes. They will perform esophageal dilatation on me because my esophagus is narrow.

Nurse: Well, do you have any questions about it? I can explain it to you.

Li Ming: Thank you very much. I just want to know whether

I will feel very painful during the operation.

Nurse: Don't worry. It causes minimal trauma and pain.

Li Ming: I see. Thanks a lot.

Nurse: You're welcome.

　　李明 3 年前被诊断为食管癌，目前进食及吞咽困难，经检查发现食管狭窄，计划明天手术。

　　护士： 早上好，李明，你今天感觉怎么样？

　　李明： 还可以。

　　护士： 你手术安排在明天，医生告诉你了吗？

　　李明： 是的，我是食管狭窄，他们要给我做扩张手术。

　　护士： 是的，你对手术还有什么疑问吗？我可以给你解释。

　　李明： 非常谢谢你，我想知道手术会很疼吗？

　　护士： 不用担心，这个手术具有创伤小、疼痛小等优点。

　　李明： 我明白了，谢谢你。

　　护士： 不客气。

第四章 胃早癌
Chapter 4　Early-stage gastric cancer

1. 了解内镜下黏膜剥离术
2. 掌握术后饮食宣教
3. 掌握以下词汇

early-stage gastric cancer　早期胃癌
endoscopic ultrasonography　超声内镜
be appropriate for　适合
endoscopic submucosal dissection　内镜黏膜下剥离术（ESD）
semi-fluid diet　半流质饮食

Li Bo is a patient in bed #29. He has been diagnosed with early-stage gastric cancer in a physical exam arranged by his company. He comes to the hospital for further treatment. Xu Dan is his primary nurse. She is talking with Li Bo and giving him a health instruction.

Xu Dan: Good morning, Li Bo. How was your sleep last night?

Li Bo: Morning, Xu Dan. I was quite worried and didn't sleep well last night. I am afraid my condition will get worse.

Xu Dan: Take it easy. You will undergo the endoscopic ultrasonography tomorrow. I am here to tell you about the dos and don'ts before the operation.

Li Bo: OK. I have undergone this examination before, and I know that I cannot eat or drink anything before the procedure.

Xu Dan: That's right. You are required to avoid food and drink after 10 pm today, until your doctor allows you. This examination helps determine whether the endoscopic submucosal dissection (ESD) is suitable for your conditions.

Li Bo: What is ESD?

Xu Dan: Generally speaking, ESD is a surgery of dissecting the lesion in your stomach using gastroscopy. Take it easy and have trust in us, since the success rate of ESD in our hospital is quite high. In addition, you need to cooperate with the nurses, and we will always be here with you.

Li Bo: Okay, thanks. What should I do after the operation?

Xu Dan: You should avoid food within the 24 hours after the procedure. After that, you may firstly choose liquid diet, like rice soup and juice, etc. When the condition gets improved, you can eat semi-liquid diet such as porridge and noodles. After recovery you can switch to regular diet, but still avoid overeating.

Li Bo: OK. Thank you very much, Xu Dan. I will keep your advice in mind!

李博是 29 床患者，体检时发现胃早癌，为进一步治疗来医院。徐丹是他的责任护士，她正在和李博对话并对他进行健康教育。

　　徐丹： 早上好李博！昨天晚上睡得怎么样？

李博：早上好！我很紧张，昨天晚上也没睡好。我怕我的病情会恶化。

徐丹：放轻松，不要紧张！明天你就要做超声内镜，我给你讲一下手术前要注意些什么吧！

李博：好的。我曾做过这个检查，知道手术前不能吃东西，也不能喝水。

徐丹：对的，你今天晚上 10 点起就要禁食、水了，直到医生说你可以吃东西了才行。这个检查主要是为了确定你的情况适不适合进行 ESD。

李博：什么是 ESD 啊？

徐丹：简而言之，ESD 就是内镜下黏膜剥离术，也就是把胃里的病灶切掉。放轻松，我们医院这类手术的成功率挺高的，要相信我们医生，另外也要配合我们的护理工作，我们会一直陪伴在你的身边！

李博：好的，谢谢你！手术后我需要注意些什么？

徐丹：术后 24 小时不能进食。之后你开始可以吃流质，像米汤、果汁之类的；病情好转后就可以吃粥、面条之类的半流质；病情恢复后才可以进普食，但还是不能暴饮暴食！

李博：好的，非常感谢你徐丹！我会牢记你的意见！

第五章 ESD/EMR 围手术期护理

Chapter 5　Perioperative care of ESD/EMR

1. 了解 ESD/EMR 围手术期护理
2. 掌握 ESD/EMR 常见并发症及判断处置
3. 掌握以下词汇

accident　意外事件　　　　　irritability　烦躁，亢奋

anti-inflammatory　抗炎　　　complication　并发症

Zhang Yi is a patient in bed #36. He has gastric stromal tumor and will undergo endoscopic submucosal dissection (ESD) tomorrow. Sun Yue is his primary nurse. She is talking with Zhang Yi and giving him a health instruction.

Sun Yue: Hello, Zhang Yi. You will undergo operation tomorrow, and I am here to tell you about what you should do before it.

Zhang Yi: Ok, I am quite worried right now. I have some questions. What procedure do I have to go through tomorrow? And what should I pay attention to?

Sun Yue: Just relax. I will explain it to you in detail. We have completed relevant examinations for you, such as chest X-ray, abdominal ultrasound, blood routine, blood coagulation and other exams and tests, all of which turn out to be normal. For now, you need to stop eating after 8 pm, and stop drinking after 10 pm. After the procedure, of course, you still can't eat anything until the doctor allows you to.

Zhang Yi: Is there any possibility for accident during the operation?

Sun Yue: First, you should trust your doctor. ESD is an safe and effective endoscopic procedure to remove gastrointestinal stromal tumors (GISTs). After the operation, you still need to avoid food and have a good rest in bed. We will monitor your blood pressure, pulse, respiration, blood oxygen saturation and other vital signs, and provide intravenous therapies such as acid suppressing, nutritional support and other infusion treatments.

If you have abdominal pain, stomach discomfort, irritability and other conditions, tell me right away. Bleeding and perforation are the main complications of this operation. It can be cured by treatment in the early phase. Second, just relax yourself. Excessive tension can also cause abdominal discomfort.

Zhang Yi: Okay. So, what else do I need to do after the operation?

Sun Yue: In short, avoid food, rest, relax, and take medication. If you need help, just let me know.

Zhang Yi: Ok. Thank you. I will keep your words in mind.

张毅是 36 床患者，患胃间质瘤，明天要做 ESD。孙悦是

他的责任护士，正在和他对话并给予他关于手术的健康宣教。

孙悦：嗨，张毅，明天你就要做手术了，我来告诉你在手术之前要做些什么。

张毅：好的，但我现在很紧张。我有几个问题：我明天要做什么手术，我需要注意什么？

孙悦：不要紧张，我会逐一向你解答。首先，我们已经给你完善了相关检查，如 X 线胸片、腹部 B 超、血常规、凝血功能等检查。目前，这些检查均无异常。你现在需要做的是今晚 8 点以后禁食，10 点以后禁水。当然，术后仍需要禁食，直到医生告知开放饮食。

张毅：手术会有什么意外吗？

孙悦：首先你应该相信医生。ESD 治疗胃间质瘤是安全且有效的，我们会严密观察你的情况。术后你仍需要禁食，绝对卧床休息，我们会监测你的血压、脉搏、呼吸、血氧饱和度等生命体征，同时给予抗炎、抑酸、营养支持等输液治疗。

如果你有腹痛、腹部不适、烦躁等情况及时告诉我。出血和穿孔是这个手术主要的并发症，但早期发现，积极地对症治疗后可以治愈。其次，你需要放松，过度紧张也会导致腹部不适。

张毅：好的，手术结束后，我还需要配合做什么？

孙悦：简而言之，禁食、休息、放松、配合用药，有情况及时告知我。

张毅：好的，谢谢。我会记住你说的话。

第六章　消化性溃疡

Chapter 6　Peptic ulcer

1. 了解疾病的主要症状
2. 了解疾病的治疗过程
3. 预防并发症的发作
4. 掌握饮食指导，药物宣教
5. 掌握以下词汇

periodic　周期性的
rhythmic　节律性的
hematemesis　呕血
melena　黑便
endoscopic hemostasis　内镜下止血
proton pump inhibitor　质子泵抑制剂
gastric mucosal protective agent　胃黏膜保护剂

Zhao Jun in bed #22 has severe peptic ulcer. He experiences frequent upper abdominal pain together with periodic and rhythmic episodes of acid reflux and hernia. He has had hematemesis and melena recently. He is now receiving treatment in hospital. Song Man is his primary nurse. She is talking with Zhao Jun and giving him a health instruction.

Song Man: Good morning, Zhao Jun. How was your sleep last night?

Zhao Jun: Good morning, Song Man. I had black stool again last night. I am quite worried. Could you tell me about the next treatment plan?

Song Man: Ok. First, the doctor will perform a gastroscopy on you to identify the area of bleeding. Then endoscopic hemostasis is given to stop bleeding based on the specific condition. Finally, proton pump inhibitor and gastric mucosal protective agents will be used to ensure better therapeutic effects.

Zhao Jun: Ok, I see. So, what else do I need to pay attention to after discharge?

Song Man: After discharge, you need to have a good rest and avoid getting too tired. Keep a regular diet and eat easily digestible food like noodles. Avoid spicy, salty food, strong tea and coffee. Take the medication on time and pay attention to your stool. In case you notice melena, come to hospital and seek medical help right away.

Zhao Jun: Ok. Thank you, Song Man. I will pay more attention.

22 床患者赵俊，他有严重的消化性溃疡。他经常出现上腹部疼痛，并周期性、节律性发作，伴有反酸、嗳气症状，最近又出现呕血和黑便。他正在医院接受治疗，宋曼是他的责任护士，她正在和赵俊对话，给他做健康教育。

宋曼： 早上好，赵俊！昨晚休息的还好吧？

赵俊： 早上好，宋曼！我昨晚又解了一次黑便，我很担心，你能告诉我接下来的治疗方案吗？

宋曼：好的。首先，医生会给你做胃镜检查，查明出血的部位。然后，根据具体情况，进行内镜下止血。最后，用抑酸药和胃黏膜保护剂来巩固治疗。

赵俊：好的，我明白了。我出院后还需要注意些什么？

宋曼：出院后，你要多注意休息，不要太劳累；进食要规律，选择易消化的食物，如面食；避免辛辣、过咸及浓茶、咖啡等；按时吃药；关注大便情况，如果出现解黑便，需要立即至医院就诊。

赵俊：好的，谢谢你，宋曼。我会多加注意的。

第七章　肝硬化
Chapter 7　Cirrhosis

 •

1. 三腔二囊管的应用
2. 饮食指导
3. 腹水监测
4. 掌握以下词汇

ascites　腹水
varices　静脉曲张（varix 的复数）
massive digestive tract bleeding　消化道大出血
Sengstaken-Blakemore tube　三腔二囊管
in terms of　就……而言
abdominal circumference　腹围

　　Qiao Kai has been diagnosed with liver cirrhosis, ascites, and esophageal and gastric varices. During hospitalization, he had massive digestive tract bleeding and now his condition has stabilized. He will be discharged from the hospital in a few days. But he is still worried, and talks to the nurse about his feeling.

　　Nurse: Good morning, Qiao Kai. Is there anything bothering you these days?

　　Qiao Kai: Yes, my doctor told me that I could go home soon.

　　Nurse: That's great. What are you worried about?

Qiao Kai: I am worried about another bleeding and other possible bad things.

Nurse: Take it easy. Do you remember the Sengstaken-Blakemore tube used for your bleeding last time? It is particularly designed for esophageal and gastric varices bleeding. Certainly, you can also take some measures to prevent bleeding.

Qiao Kai: But I do not know what I should do, particularly in terms of my diet.

Nurse: You'd better eat soft, meshed and easily digestible food. Avoid irritating food such as raw and hard food, fried food, and avoid strong tea and alcohol too. Furthermore, stay away from hot food.

Qiao Kai: I see. My doctor has also told me to measure abdominal circumference and weight every day.

Nurse: Sure, it is very important to monitor ascites.

Qiao Kai: Thank you. I feel more relaxed now.

Nurse: You're welcome.

患者乔凯诊断为肝硬化、腹水、食管胃底静脉曲张。他在住院期间曾发生过一次消化道大出血，现在病情已经稳定，再过几天就可以出院了，但是他仍很担心，并告诉了护士。

护士：早上好，乔凯，这几天有什么事情困扰你吗?

乔凯：是的，我的医生告诉我很快就可以出院了。

护士：这是个好消息啊，你担心什么?

乔凯：我怕再次出血，或者出现其他不好的情况。

护士：不用担心，你还记得你上次出血时用的那根三腔二囊管吗？那是专门为食管胃底静脉曲张出血而设计的，当然，你也可以采取一些措施预防出血。

乔凯：但我不知道应该做什么，尤其是饮食上需要注意什么？

护士：你应该进食软的、易嚼的、容易消化的食物，生硬食物、油炸食物之类刺激性的食物不要吃，不要饮浓茶和酒，同时避免进食过热的食物。

乔凯：我明白了，医生还要求我每天测量腹围和体重。

护士：是的，监测腹水很重要。

乔凯：谢谢你，我现在放松了很多。

护士：不客气。

第八章 胆管结石

Chapter 8　Cholangiolithiasis

学习目标

1. 了解疾病的主要症状
2. 了解疾病的治疗过程
3. 预防并发症的发作
4. 掌握饮食指导，药物宣教
5. 掌握以下词汇

　jaundice　黄疸
　antibiotic　抗生素
　suppurative cholecystitis　化脓性胆囊炎
　collaborate with　与…合作
　high protein　高蛋白质

Li Bo received ERCP treatment yesterday for cholangiolithiasis accompanied by abdominal pain, fever, and yellowing of the skin. Jin Chen is his primary nurse. She is talking with Li Bo and giving him a health instruction.

Jin Chen: Good morning, Li Bo! It is a nice day today. Did you have a good rest last night?

Li Bo: Good morning, Jin Chen! I'm sorry that I did not follow your advice and drank a glass of water yesterday. Now I feel painful in the upper abdomen and have a high temperature.

Jin Chen: You should avoid food after ERCP. We will

provide sufficient fluid replacement treatment and proper antibiotics to prevent postoperative pyogenic cholangitis according to your doctor's advice. To make sure you recover soon, please follow our advice.

Li Bo: Sorry, Jin Chen. I understand and will fully collaborate with the doctor, but I am still worried about my condition after discharge.

Jin Chen: Take it easy. Choose proper diet, eat small but frequent meals, and eat low-fat, high-protein, easily digestible, high-vitamin, and dietary fiber-rich food. Never skip breakfast. Keep a balance between work and rest, and come back for regular outpatient follow-up.

Li Bo: Ok, thank you very much. I will do what you have advised.

患者李博因胆结石伴有腹部疼痛、发热、皮肤发黄症状，昨天行 ERCP 治疗。金晨是他的责任护士，正在和李博对话，并进行健康教育。

金晨： 早安，李博，今天天气很好，你昨晚休息的怎么样？

李博： 早安，金晨，对不起，我没有遵循你的建议，偷偷喝了一杯水，现在感觉上腹部疼痛，体温也有点上升了。

金晨： ERCP 后你需要进行严格的禁食、禁水，我们会遵医嘱给你进行补液治疗，并使用适当的抗生素，预防术后化脓性胆管炎的发作。为了你能尽快康复，请配合我们。

李博： 对不起，金晨，我知道了，我会全力配合你们的治疗，可是我还是比较担心出院以后的情况。

金晨：别紧张。选择适当的饮食，少餐多餐，吃低脂肪、高蛋白质、易消化、高维生素、富含膳食纤维的食物，不能不吃早餐。劳逸结合，定期进行门诊随访。

李博：好的，真的太感谢你了，我会认真听从你的建议。

第九章 肝癌

Chapter 9 Hepatic carcinoma

 •·····································

1. 了解肝癌的不同治疗方法
2. 熟悉 TACE 手术路径及术后注意事项
3. 掌握以下词汇

> hepatic cell carcinoma 肝细胞癌（HCC）
> transcatheter arterial chemoembolization (TACE)
>   经导管动脉化疗栓塞
> radiofrequency ablation 射频消融

Zhang Jun is a patient who has been diagnosed with hepatic carcinoma (HCC). He comes to the hospital for transcatheter arterial chemoembolization (TACE) and radiofrequency ablation. After the operation, he returns to the ward. Xiao Ran is his primary nurse. She is talking with Zhang Jun and giving him a health instruction.

Xiao Ran: Hello, Zhang Jun, how are you feeling?

Zhang Jun: Hello, Xiao Ran. I am a little worried. Could you tell me what TACE and radiofrequency ablation are?

Xiao Ran: All right, take it easy. There are currently two kinds of TACE combined with thermal ablation. ① Sequential ablation. One to four weeks after TACE treatment, additional radiofrequency ablation will be performed. ② Synchronized ablation. During TACE treatment, radiofrequency or microwave ablation can significantly improve the clinical efficacy and reduce liver function damage. TACE takes advantage of the fact that HCC is mainly supplied by the hepatic artery. By injecting chemotherapeutic drugs and embolization materials into the blood supplying artery of the tumor, the purpose of tumor ischemic necrosis and local drug chemotherapy can be achieved. It has the advantages of good therapeutic effect, minimal trauma, repeatable treatment, etc., and is the preferred choice for treating mid to late-stage liver cancer.

Zhang Jun: Can you tell me what I should pay attention to after operation?

Xiao Ran: OK, Zhang Jun. After the operation, you should monitor your temperature. Take good care of oral cavity. Fever after TACE is common, but infectious complications are rare. It is usually a result of tumor necrosis and collateral damage to normal liver tissue. When the body temperature exceeds 39.0°C or the fever lasts for more than one week, anti-infective treatment will be required.

Zhang Jun: Thank you very much, Xiao Ran. I will keep your advice in mind.

张军是肝癌患者，他来到医院行经导管动脉化疗栓塞及射频消融术，术后安全返回病房，小冉是他的责任护士，她正在和张军对话并进行健康宣教。

小冉：你好，张军，感觉怎样？

张军：你好，小冉！我有些紧张。你能再解释一下经导管动脉化疗栓塞术（TACE）和射频消融术是什么吗？

小冉：好的，你不要太紧张，目前有两种 TACE 联合热消融治疗方式。① 序贯消融：先行 TACE 治疗，术后 1～4 周内加用射频或微波消融。② 同步消融：在 TACE 治疗时，同时给予射频或微波消融，可以明显提高临床疗效，并减轻肝功能损伤。TACE 利用肝癌主要由肝动脉供血的特点，通过向肿瘤供血动脉注入化疗药物和栓塞材料，达到肿瘤缺血坏死和局部药物化疗的目的，具有疗效好、创伤小、可重复治疗等优点，是目前中晚期肝癌首选的治疗方法。

张军：你能告诉我，术后我要注意些什么？

小冉：好的，张军，术后你要监测体温，做好口腔护理，术后会出现肿瘤组织、坏死重吸收而致的吸收热。当体温超过 39.0℃，或发热持续 1 周以上时，需要进行抗感染治疗。

张军：非常感谢你，小冉！我会牢记你的建议。

第十章 慢性胰腺炎

Chapter 10　Chronic pancreatitis

学习目标 •--------------------------------

1. 慢性胰腺炎疼痛的原因
2. 如何缓解慢性胰腺炎疼痛
3. 掌握以下词汇

> intermittent　间歇的；间断的
> upper abdominal pain　上腹痛
> diarrhea　腹泻
> pancreatic duct hypertension　胰管高压
> analgesic　止痛剂；止痛的
> extracorporeal shock wave lithotripsy (ESWL)　体外冲击波碎石术

Zhang Jun suffers from intermittent upper abdominal pain for two years accompanied by diarrhea and weight loss. The pain has been getting worse recently. The purpose of this hospitalization is to manage the pain. Xiao Ran is his primary nurse. They are having a conversation.

Xiao Ran: Good morning, Zhang Jun. Did you have a good sleep last night?

Zhang Jun: Good morning, Xiao Ran. I did not sleep well last night. The pain has been bothering me and kept me awake.

Xiao Ran: I am sorry to hear that.

Zhang Jun: Xiao Ran, why is chronic pancreatitis painful?

Xiao Ran: Abdominal pain caused by chronic pancreatitis is mainly the result of pancreatic duct hypertension, or increased pancreatic parenchyma/interstitial tension. The other major cause could be peripancreatic and celiac plexus inflammation.

Zhang Jun: Oh, I see. How to deal with it?

Xiao Ran: First, avoid alcohol, quit smoking, and choose proper diet. Second, use medications such as pancreatic enzyme supplementation, antioxidant, somatostatin and analgesic. Third, ESWL treatment may also help to remove stones and reduce pain.

Zhang Jun: Ok, thank you.

Xiao Ran: You're welcome. Wish you a speedy recovery.

　　患者张军有间歇性上腹部疼痛，反复持续 2 年，伴腹泻、体重下降，最近疼痛症状加重，这次住院的目的是控制疼痛，小冉是他的责任护士，他们正在交谈。

　　小冉： 早上好，张军，昨晚休息得怎样？

　　张军： 早上好，小冉，我昨晚睡得很不好，疼痛一直困扰着我，使我难以入睡。

　　小冉： 很抱歉听到这些。

　　张军： 小冉，慢性胰腺炎为什么会疼痛？

　　小冉： 慢性胰腺炎引起腹痛的原因主要为胰管高压，胰腺实质／间质张力升高；另一个主要原因可能是胰腺周围和腹腔神经丛炎症。

张军：哦，我明白了。如何处理呢？

小冉：首先要禁酒、戒烟、控制饮食，其次要用药物治疗，包括胰酶制剂、抗氧化剂、生长抑素及止痛药的应用。此外，体外冲击波碎石术也有助于清除结石及缓解疼痛。

张军：好的，谢谢你。

小冉：不客气，祝你早日康复。

第十一章　体外冲击波碎石围手术期护理
Chapter 11　Perioperative care of ESWL

1. ESWL 前准备
2. ESWL 术后注意事项
3. 掌握以下词汇

    indwelling infusion needle　留置针
    intravenous anesthesia　静脉麻醉
    nursing assistant　护工
    blood amylase　血淀粉酶
    abdominal symptoms　腹部症状

Zhang Jun is a patient with pancreatic duct stones. He needs to undergo extracorporeal shock wave lithotripsy (ESWL). Xiao Ran is his primary nurse. She is talking with the patient and giving him a health instruction.

Xiao Ran: Good morning, Zhang Jun.

Zhang Jun: Good morning, Xiao Ran.

Xiao Ran: According to your condition, the doctor has made a treatment plan for you and will perform ESWL for you tomorrow.

Zhang Jun: Okay, what preparations do I need to make?

Xiao Ran: Before ESWL, you should understand the preparation for the operation, which is performed under general anesthesia. You should keep a happy mood and have a good rest the day before the operation. If you cannot fall asleep, call the doctor, who will prescribe you sleep medication. Avoid eating and drinking 8 hours before the operation. We will place an indwelling infusion needle for you tomorrow morning before the operation, so that you can have intravenous anesthesia before the lithotripsy operation. Nursing assistant will take you to the endoscopy center. You will need a family member to accompany you.

Zhang Jun: Okay, thank you.

Xiao Ran: After ESWL, you need to rest in bed. The recovery of consciousness will be under close watch. We will also monitor your heart rate, blood pressure, respiration, pulse, urine and stool colors, and other discomfort symptoms. Blood amylase will be tested 3 hours and 24 hours after the operation. You need to fast for 24 hours and when to resume meals depends on the level of blood amylase and abdominal symptoms.

Zhang Jun: Ok, I will certainly do what the operation requires.

Xiao Ran: Come on! Let's more forward together.

 译文

张军是一位胰管结石患者，需要做体外冲击波碎石，小冉是他的责任护士，她正在和患者对话，并进行健康宣教。

小冉： 早上好，张军。

张军： 早上好，小冉。

小冉： 根据你的病情，医生为你制订了治疗方案，将在明天为你做体外冲击波碎石术。

张军：好的，我需要准备什么？

小冉：体外冲击波碎石术是在全麻状态下进行，你需要先了解下术前的注意事项。手术前一天要保持愉悦的心情，保证良好的休息。如果睡不着，可以告知医生，医生会给你开助睡眠的药物，术前常规禁食、禁饮 8 小时。明天早上手术前我们会为你留置一个静脉输液留置针，这样方便你在碎石手术前进行静脉麻醉，让你无痛苦地进行碎石手术。明天会有专人来接你去内镜中心，需要有一名家属陪着你。

张军：好的，谢谢。

小冉：术后，你需要卧床休息，我们会观察你神志恢复情况，监测心率、血压、呼吸、脉搏，观察大小便颜色及其他不适症状，监测术后 3 小时、24 小时血淀粉酶。你将禁食 24 小时，根据血淀粉酶水平和腹部症状决定何时进食。

张军：好的，我一定会配合的。

小冉：加油！我们一起努力。

第十二章　急性胰腺炎

Chapter 12　Acute pancreatitis

学习目标

1. 急性胰腺炎定义、症状和诊断
2. 急性胰腺炎的治疗原则
3. 掌握以下词汇

abdominal bloating	腹胀	significant	显著的
waist and back pain	腰背部 疼痛	mirabilite	芒硝
		rhubarb	大黄

Zhang Jun is an ICU patient diagnosed with acute pancreatitis. He had epigastric pain, abdominal bloating, together with waist and back pain for one day after drinking at a dinner. Xiao Ran is his primary nurse. She is talking with Zhang Jun.

Xiao Ran: Hi, Zhang Jun, how are you feeling now? Is your abdominal pain getting better?

Zhang Jun: No, I feel awful, with terrible pain in my abdomen. What's wrong with me?

Xiao Ran: I have to tell you that you have acute pancreatitis. It is an inflammation of the pancreas and surrounding tissues. It is caused by the activation of pancreatic enzymes in the pancreas. Clinical manifestations include acute epigastric pain, nausea, vomiting, fever, and significantly increased amylase in blood and urine.

Zhang Jun: Oh, how can I relieve the abdominal distention and pain?

Xiao Ran: Clinical data has confirmed that rhubarb enema combined with mirabilite external application can effectively alleviate abdominal distension and pain. Rhubarb increases the secretion of bile. As a laxative, it promotes intestinal peristalsis, eliminates intestinal inflammatory factors and protects gastrointestinal mucosal barrier. Mirabilite external application can absorb peritoneal exudates, relieve inflammation and pain, prevent infection, improve local microcirculation, and promote the recovery of gastrointestinal function.

Zhang Jun: Thank you. How is acute pancreatitis treated?

Xiao Ran: Treatments for acute pancreatitis include dry fasting, effective fluid resuscitation, maintenance of water and electrolyte balance, nutritional support, anti-infection treatment, and prevention of local and systemic complications. The most effective treatment is early and effective fluid resuscitation. Early inflammation can cause blood capillary leakage, leading to insufficient blood circulation. Effective liquid resuscitation helps to maintain blood volume, ensure the pancreas microcirculation perfusion, and further prevent local and systemic complications, such as pancreatic necrosis, systemic inflammatory response syndrome and multiple organ failures.

Zhang Jun: This sounds serious and I am quite worried.

Xiao Ran: Take it easy. Acute pancreatitis itself is not scary. What's terrible is the late complications. If you follow the treatment plan, you will get well soon.

Zhang Jun: Ok, I will do what you said.

Xiao Ran: Come on! Let's work together to conquer the disease.

住在 ICU 的张军是一位急性胰腺炎患者，聚餐饮酒后上腹痛、腹胀伴腰背部疼痛 1 天，被诊断为急性胰腺炎，小冉是他的责任护士，正在和张军交流。

小冉：嗨，张军，现在感觉怎么样，腹痛症状有缓解吗？

张军：没有，我感觉糟糕透了，腹部胀痛得厉害，我得了什么病？

小冉：我很抱歉地告诉你，你得了急性胰腺炎。急性胰腺炎是多种病因导致胰酶在胰腺内被激活后，引起胰腺及其周围组织自身消化、水肿、出血甚至坏死的炎症反应。临床以急性上腹痛、恶心、呕吐、发热和血 / 尿淀粉酶明显升高等为特点。

张军：哦，怎样才能缓解腹部胀痛呢？

小冉：临床数据证实，中药大黄灌肠联合芒硝外敷能有效缓解腹部胀痛，大黄具有利胆、泻下、促进肠道蠕动、清除肠道内炎症因子、保护胃肠道黏膜屏障；芒硝外敷具有吸收腹腔渗液、消炎镇痛、预防感染、改善局部微循环、促进与恢复消化道功能等功效。

张军：谢谢，急性胰腺炎应该怎么治疗呢？

小冉：急性胰腺炎的治疗措施包括禁食、禁水、有效的液体复苏、维持水电解质平衡、营养支持、抗感染治疗、防治局部及全身并发症。最有效的治疗是早期有效的液体复苏，炎症反应会引起毛细血管渗漏，导致循环血量不足，有效的液体复苏能维持血容量，保证了胰腺的微循环灌注，进一步防止局部和全身并发症的发生，如胰腺坏死、全身炎症反应综合征以及多器官功能衰竭。

张军：听起来很严重，我很担心。

小冉：不用担心，急性胰腺炎本身不可怕，可怕的是后期并发症，如果好好配合治疗，相信你很快就能好起来的。

张军：好的，我一定按照你说的做。

小冉：加油！我们一起努力战胜疾病。

第十三章　胰腺癌

Chapter 13　Pancreatic cancer

 学习目标 •

1. 胰腺癌的主要治疗方式
2. 支架植入的手术途径
3. 支架植入术后的注意事项
4. 掌握以下词汇

massage　按摩	significant pain　明显的疼痛
strenuous exercise　剧烈运动	bile ducts　胆管
treatment plan　治疗计划	jaundice　黄疸

Xiao Rui is a patient in bed #20. She was diagnosed with pancreatic cancer a week ago and is waiting for treatment in hospital now. Su Shan is her primary nurse. She is talking with the patient.

Su Shan: Morning, Xiao Rui. How are you feeling today?

Xiao Rui: Morning, Su Shan. Just as usual. You know, I'm not feeling well recently. Is there any better treatment plan?

Su Shan: The treatments for pancreatic cancer are surgery, implantation of I^{125} seeds or stent under the guidance of endoscope.

Xiao Rui: What should I pay attention to after the operation?

Su Shan: There are precautions after placing stent. To prevent the detachment or dislocation of stent, you should not massage your abdomen and should avoid strenuous exercise.

Besides, keep off cold food or the food with coarse fiber. In case of abdominal pain after discharge, you need to seek medical attention immediately.

Xiao Rui: Thank you for your detailed explanation. And I have one more question — why do I feel no pain? Pancreatic cancer is known to cause severe pain.

Su Shan: You are right, that's a very professional question. Most people know that pancreatic cancer is the most lethal tumor causing intolerable pain. From a professional viewpoint, we need to identify the location of the tumor. If the tumor is in the tail of the pancreas, close to the posterior peritoneal plexus, the patient may feel significant pain. If the tumor is in the head or neck of the pancreas, it can block the bile ducts, the pancreatic ducts, even the duodenum, and the patient may have difficulty eating, accompanied by jaundice and other symptoms.

Xiao Rui: I see. My tumor is in the body of the pancreas, so I feel less painful. Thank you for your explanation.

　　小蕊是 20 床患者，确诊胰腺癌 1 周，目前在医院等待治疗方案。苏珊是她的责任护士，正在与她交流。

　　苏珊：早上好，小蕊，今天觉得怎么样？

　　小蕊：早上好，苏珊，还是老样子，你知道我最近不太舒服，没有更好的治疗方案吗？

　　苏珊：胰腺癌的治疗方案主要有外科手术治疗、内镜下植入 I^{125} 放射性粒子或胰管支架。

小蕊：我手术后需要注意些什么？

苏珊：放置支架后有一些注意事项。为了预防支架的脱落或移位，首先要避免剧烈运动和按摩腹部，其次不可以进食过冷的食物，同时也要避免进食粗纤维。如果出院后你有腹痛的话，需要及时到医院就诊。

小蕊：谢谢你详细的解释。我还有一个问题，为何我感觉不到疼痛。你知道，胰腺癌是以疼痛著称的。

苏珊：是的，你的问题很专业。很多人都知道胰腺癌是癌中之王，疼痛难忍。从专业的角度，我们要评估肿瘤的位置。如果肿瘤位于胰腺尾部，靠近后腹膜神经丛，患者的疼痛会很明显；如果肿瘤在胰腺头颈部，它会阻塞胆管、胰管甚至十二指肠，患者可能有进食困难，同时伴有黄疸和其他症状。

小蕊：我明白了，我的肿瘤是在胰腺体部，所以我的感觉较轻，谢谢你的解释。

第十四章　炎症性肠病

Chapter 14　Inflammatory bowel disease

 学习目标

1. 了解疾病中对排便的观察
2. 掌握饮食指导及保留灌肠的注意事项
3. 掌握以下词汇

bloody purulent stool　脓血便	retention enema　保留灌肠
left lower abdomen　左下腹	left lateral decubitus　左侧卧位
barbecue　烧烤，烤肉	sigmoid colon　乙状结肠

Wang Ming in bed #25 is a patient diagnosed with inflammatory bowel disease. He has had recurrent bloody purulent stool for 2 years. The symptoms have worsened recently, with bowel movements occurring 4 to 9 times a day, accompanied by dull pain in the lower left abdomen and no fever. Wang fang is his primary nurse. She is talking with Wang Ming and giving him a health instruction.

Wang Fang: Good morning, Wang Ming. It is a nice day today. You don't look very well, what's up?

Wang Ming: Thank you for your care. Yes, last night I lost control of myself. I ate some barbecue and had diarrhea later.

Wang Fang: Oh, I am so sorry to hear that. If you lose control of your mouth and stomach, it is very difficult to manage your inflammatory bowel disease. Starting from tonight, we will give you medication for retention enema as directed by the doctor.

Wang Ming: Can you tell me what food I can eat? How should I cooperate with you to preserve the enema? I will take your advice seriously this time.

Wang Fang: Ok, Wang Ming. First, you should have a good rest. I suggest you choose a diet rich in calorie, protein and vitamin, but low in residue and fat. Retention enema allows the drug to work directly on the intestinal mucosa locally, which has very good therapeutic effects. A disposable sputum suction tube will be used for enema, as it can reduce your discomfort.

Enema medication will be used at 37 to 38℃, which is closest to human gut temperature. Second, when we inject the enema solution into your body, the volume will not exceed 200 mL each time, so that you won't feel like going to the bathroom, which serves the purpose of retention enema. In addition, when we perform enema, you need to maintain a left lateral decubitus position, so that the medication can directly reach the sigmoid colon. Finally, you need to go to the bathroom before enema is applied, so that the retention time will be longer.

Wang Ming: Ok, thank you so much. I will keep your advice in mind.

　　25 床王明是一位炎症性肠病患者，他反复出现黏液性血便 2 年，近来症状加重，大便每日达 4～9 次，伴有左下腹隐痛，无发热，他来到医院，王芳是他的责任护士，她正在对王明进行健康教育。

王芳：早上好，王明，今天是美好的一天，我看你今天气色有点不太好，怎么了？

王明：谢谢你的关心，是的，昨晚我实在是没忍住，吃了点烧烤，后面就腹泻。

王芳：哦，我很抱歉听这些，如果你没办法管住你的嘴和胃，那么很难控制你的炎症性肠病。从今天晚上开始，我们将遵医嘱对你进行药物保留灌肠。

王明：你能不能告诉我什么食物能吃。我应该如何配合你们进行保留灌肠呢？这次我一定认真听从你的意见。

王芳：好的，王明，首先你要保持良好的休息，我建议你多吃高热量、高蛋白质、高维生素、少渣少油饮食，保留灌肠可以使药物直接作用于局部肠道，具有良好的治疗效果。首先在选择灌肠器械的时候我们会选择一次性吸痰管，这样可以减轻你的不适感。使用 37～38℃的灌肠药物，这样最接近人体肠道温度。其次在给你注入灌肠液的时候一次不能超过 200 mL，这样不会使你产生便意，以达到保留灌肠的目的。我们在灌肠的时候你要保持左侧卧位，这样可以使药物直接到达乙状结肠，最后希望你灌肠前去下卫生间，这样灌肠液保留的时间将会更持久。

王明：好的，非常感谢你，我会认真牢记你的建议。

第十五章 肠息肉

Chapter 15　Intestinal polyps

 学习目标

1. 了解肠息肉术后需要观察什么
2. 肠息肉术后容易发生什么并发症，如何预防
3. 掌握饮食指导、药物宣教
4. 掌握以下词汇

complication　并发症	spicy food　辛辣食物
precaution　预防措施	oral anticoagulants　口服抗凝药
perforation　穿孔	coronary heart disease　冠心病
porridge　粥	pathological report　病理报告

Wang Fang is a patient in bed #26 who has been found to have colon polyps during in a health check up. She was admitted to the hospital and received routine treatment before undergoing endoscopic polypectomy. The patient has returned to the ward. Her primary nurse Xiao Li is talking with him and giving her instructions on preventing postoperative complications.

Xiao Li: Hello, Wang Fang. Now the procedure is over. How are you feeling?

Wang Fang: Thanks, nurse. I'm fine. Is there anything that I should pay more attention to?

Xiao Li: Within one week after discharge, please observe the appearance, color, and size of stool. Pay special attention to abdominal pain. They are the signs of bleeding or delayed perforation. It is normal to have a small amount of blood in stool. If you have a large amount of blood in stool or huge abdominal pain, get medical treatment in time.

Wang Fang: OK, thank you, nurse. Do I need to take other precautions?

Xiao Li: After operation, you should rest in bed to prevent complications such as bleeding and perforation. Try to avoid squatting and holding breath. Do not sit, stand, and walk for a long time. Avoid eating and drinking within the first 6 hours after operation. If there is no discomfort, you can eat residue-free and semi-liquid diet for 2 to 3 days. Porridge, noodles, and lotus root powder are preferred in the first week after discharge. You can also eat small portions of egg and fish. Vegetables, fruits, and clumps of indigestible food are allowed three days later. Please keep away from cigarette, alcohol, spicy, and irritating food. In addition, you may choose foods that nourish mucosa and stop bleeding, such as pear juice, lotus root juice, balsam pear, black sesame, etc. Patients should keep off oral anticoagulants or anti-platelet drugs such as aspirin for one week after operation. Drugs for hypertension, diabetes, coronary heart disease and other diseases should be taken as usual.

Wang Fang: OK, nurse, thank you very much.

Xiao Li: You're welcome. And you must stay cheerful and avoid getting angry. Irritability and depression may lead to the contraction of the intestinal mucosa and block blood flow. One week after discharge, check the pathological report of polyps. If it is benign, regular follow-up is needed. If it is malignant, please make an appointment with your doctor and discuss the subsequent treatment plan as soon as possible.

Wang Fang: Thank you so much. I will keep your words in mind.

　　王芳是 26 床患者，因体检发现肠息肉，入院后予常规对症治疗后行内镜下肠息肉摘除术，小李是她的责任护士，患者术后安全返回病房，小李护士正在做防范术后并发症宣教。

　　小李：你好，王芳，现在手术已经做完了，感觉怎么样？

　　王芳：你好，护士！我现在感觉还好，请问我以后要注意些什么？

　　小李：出院后 1 周内观察大便的性状、颜色、量及有无腹痛，及时发现有无出血或迟发性穿孔的可能。少量便血为正常表现，若出现大量便血或腹部疼痛应及时就诊。

　　王芳：好的，谢谢护士，我还有其他方面的注意事项吗？

　　小李：术后应卧床休息，以避免出血、穿孔等并发症；术后尽量避免下蹲、屏气的动作，也不宜久坐、久立、久行等。术后应禁食 24 小时，无不适继而进无渣半流质饮食 2～3 天；出院后 1 周内以稀饭、面条、藕粉类软食为主，鸡蛋、鱼肉类可少量摄取，蔬菜、水果、团块状难消化食物 3 天后摄取，禁忌烟酒、辛辣刺激食物。另外，多吃一些可以营养黏膜、通便止血的食物比较好，如梨汁、藕汁、苦瓜、黑芝麻等。有口服抗凝血药物或抗血小板药物如阿司匹林的患者术后应停药 1 周，除此之外的高血压、糖尿病、冠心病等疾病所服药物应照常服用。

王芳：好的，护士，太感谢了！

小李：不客气，还有你一定要保持心情开朗，勿郁怒动火，心境不宽、烦躁忧郁会使肠黏膜收缩，血行不畅。出院 1 周后应关注息肉病理报告，如为良性需定期复查，如为恶性应来门诊随访决定下一步治疗方案，切勿耽误病情的治疗。

王芳：非常感谢你，我会牢记你的话。

第十六章 胶囊内镜检查

Chapter 16   Capsule endoscopy

 学习目标

1. 了解胶囊内镜的检查方法
2. 熟悉胶囊内镜的适应证
3. 掌握胶囊内镜检查期间的注意事项
4. 掌握以下词汇

magnetic field   磁场   obscure   不明原因的

Li Bo has had obscure gastrointestinal bleeding symptoms for three months. He comes to the hospital for further examination. Lin Yun is his primary nurse. She is talking with Li Bo.

Lin Yun: Good morning, Li Bo. How are you feeling today?

Li Bo: Morning, Lin Yun. I am not feeling well. My stool is still black. I am a little worried about it. Do you have any corresponding examinations?

Lin Yun: Yes, you can try a capsule endoscopy. You just need to take a capsule. It will go down your digestive tract and takes photos. Then we can see clearly what is happening in the digestive tract.

Li Bo: That is great. What should I do?

Lin Yun: Well, here are some tips for you. Avoid food or drink after 10 pm tonight and get prepared for bowel cleaning as required. After taking the capsule, don't exercise vigorously during the examination and stay away from the magnetic field. You may drink water two hours later. A small portion of light food is allowed four hours later.

Li Bo: Thanks a lot. I will follow your advice.

Lin Yun: Wish you a speedy recovery.

患者李博出现不明原因的消化道出血症状 3 个月了，此次为了进一步检查来我院就诊，林允是他的责任护士，她正在和李博交流。

林允：早安，李博，今天感觉如何？

李博：早安，林允。感觉不太好，我的大便依然发黑，我有些担心，有什么适合我的检查方法吗？

林允：有的，可以做胶囊内镜检查。你只需服用一颗胶囊，它就会沿着消化道一路向下，并拍摄图片。从而让我们清晰地看到消化道内情况。

李博：那真是太好了，那我需要做些什么呢？

林允：有一些需要你配合的事项。晚上 10 点以后不要吃东西或喝东西，根据要求做肠道清洁准备。胶囊吞服后，检查过程中请不要剧烈运动，并远离磁场。2 小时后可以喝水。4 小时后可以吃少量清淡的食物。

李博：非常感谢你，我会遵循你的建议。

林允：祝你早日康复！

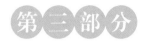

专科护理操作

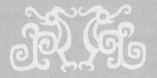

Part Three

Specialist Nursing Operations

第一章　三腔二囊管

Chapter 1　Sengstaken-Blakemore tube

---

1. 了解三腔二囊管的作用
2. 掌握三腔二囊管的使用方法及注意事项
3. 了解三腔二囊管止血的优势
4. 掌握以下词汇

liver cirrhosis　肝硬化	estimate　估算
Sengstaken-Blakemore tube 　　三腔二囊管	paraffin oil　石蜡油
	pylorus　幽门
esophageal and gastric varices 　　食管胃底静脉曲张	hemorrhage and necrosis　出血 　　和坏死
portal hypertension　门脉高压	

Li Ming is a patient diagnosed with liver cirrhosis. He is conscious with poor spirit and vomits around 500 mL of blood within a short period of time. He is using Sengstaken-Blakemore tube.

Xiao Ran is a gastroenterology nurse and Lin Yun is a newly graduated intern nurse.

Lin Yun: Miss Xiao Ran, how does the Sengstaken-Blakemore tube achieve hemostasis?

Xiao Ran: Sengstaken-Blakemore tube is used for patients with esophageal and gastric varices bleeding caused by portal hypertension.

Hemostasis is achieved through the compression of Sengstaken-Blakemore tube.

Lin Yun: How to use a Sengstaken-Blakemore tube?

Xiao Ran: First, patient cooperation is required for the purpose of rapid hemostasis. Second, check the tube before intubation. Make sure there is no leak, and the sizes and shapes of the inflated balloons are equal. After exhausting the air in the two balloons, mark stomach balloon, esophagus balloon and stomach lumen. Third, measure the distance from the patient's nose to the subxiphoid process, and estimate the insertion length. Generally, the insertion length is 55 to 65 cm. Apply paraffin oil to the anterior segment of the tube, the double balloon portion and the patient's nasal cavity. Have the patient take 20 to 30 mL paraffin oil orally. Insert the tube gently from the nostril. When it reaches the pharynx, instruct the patient to swallow. When the estimated distance is reached, if the gastric contents can be extracted from the gastric tube cavity, it indicates that the tip has reached the pylorus. Inject 200 mL air into the gastric sac, seal the open end of the gastric balloon tube by a vascular clamp, and then pull outward the tube. If hemostasis cannot be achieved, inject 80 to 100 mL air into the esophageal sac, seal the open end of the esophageal balloon tube with a vascular clamp, and continuously pull the outer end of the tube with a weight of 0.5 kg through a pulley device. The pulling direction is at a 45 degrees to the patient's supine position, so as to achieve hemostasis through air bag compression. Make a clear mark on the exposed part of the tube entering the nostril for observation. Connect the gastric tube opening to the gastrointestinal decompression device to observe hemorrhage.

Generally, Sengstaken-Blakemore tube is put in place for 12 hours. If there is no sign of second bleeding, traction may be relaxed. If bleeding continues, traction can be sustained up to 24 hours. After 24 hours, traction must be relaxed to reduce the risk of erosive hemorrhage and necrosis caused by long-time stress of esophageal and gastric fundus mucosa. Before deflation, have the patient take 20 to 30 mL of paraffin oil orally. Slowly draw out the air in the esophageal balloon. Keep monitoring the possible bleeding before exhausting air in gastric balloon. If bleeding continues, maintain the traction and compression to stop bleeding. If bleeding stops, relax the traction and keep them in place for another 24 to 48 hours. If there is no sign of second bleeding, pull out the tube and observe for at least 24 hours. If no bleeding is observed afterwards, regular diet can be restarted.

Lin Yun: Well, why not choose other quick hemostasis methods?

Xiao Ran: The vision is poor due to large amount of blood in esophageal and stomach cavity during acute hemorrhage. The success rate of emergency endoscopic hemostasis is low. However, emergency surgery is hampered by poor liver function and limited effective circulating volume. Therefore, compression hemostasis using Sengstaken-Blakemore tube is the preferred emergency treatment for patients with cirrhosis and gastrointestinal bleeding.

Lin Yun: I see. Thank you, Xiao Ran.

Xiao Ran: You're welcome.

　　李明是一位肝硬化患者，神志清、精神不振，短时间内呕吐出鲜血量约 500 mL，正在使用三腔二囊管止血。

　　小冉是一名消化科护士，林允是一名刚毕业的实习护士。

　　林允：小冉老师，三腔二囊管是怎么达到止血目的？

　　小冉：三腔二囊管适用于门脉高压所致的食管胃底静脉曲张破裂出血的患者，通过三腔二囊管压迫达到止血的目的。

　　林允：怎么使用三腔二囊管呢？

　　小冉：首先，取得患者配合以达到迅速止血的目的。第二，插管前先检查双气囊及三腔管是否漏气，充气后气囊大小形状是否均匀，并抽净双气囊内气体，并对胃气囊、食管气囊和胃腔进行标记。第三，测量患者鼻部至剑突下距离，估算插入长度，一般在 55～65 cm，将三腔管前段、双气囊部及患者鼻腔涂石蜡油，并让患者口服 20～30 mL 石蜡油，将三腔二囊管从鼻孔轻轻插入，到达咽部时嘱患者做吞咽动作，到达估算距离时，若能由胃管腔抽出胃内容物，表示头端已至幽门。向胃囊内注入 200 mL 空气，用血管钳封闭胃气囊管的开口端，再向外牵拉三腔二囊管；如不能有效止血，食管囊内注气80～100 mL，用血管钳封闭食管气囊管的开口端，用 0.5 kg重物通过滑车装置持续牵拉三腔二囊管外端，牵拉方向与患者平卧体位成 45°，以达到气囊压迫止血的目的。三腔二囊管露出鼻腔部分做一醒目标志，以便观察，将胃管开口连接胃肠道减压装置，观察出血情况。

　　三腔二囊管一般放置 12 小时后观察无再次出血情况，可放松牵引，若仍有出血迹象，可适当延长至 24 小时，24 小时后必须放松牵引，防止食管胃底黏膜压迫时间过长引起糜烂性出血、坏死，放气前让患者口服石蜡油 20～30 mL，缓慢抽出食管囊内气体，继续观察有无出血，再放胃囊气体。若仍有出血迹象，继续牵引压迫止血，若出血已停止，可放松牵引后继续放置 24～48 小时，若无继续出血迹象，可拔出三腔二囊管，拔管后至少观察 24 小时，仍无出血迹象，可适当恢复饮食。

林允： 嗯，为什么不选择其他快速止血方式呢？

小冉： 肝硬化患者因短时间量大出血，食管胃腔内充满血液使视野模糊不清，急诊内镜止血成功率不高。而急诊外科手术受肝功能分级分佳及有效循环血容量有限的影响，因此，三腔二囊管压迫止血是肝硬化消化道出血患者首选的紧急止血措施。

林允： 明白了，谢谢小冉。

小冉： 不客气！

第二章 鼻胆管

Chapter 2 Nasobiliary drainage tube

1. 了解鼻胆管的留置时间
2. 掌握留置鼻胆管期间的饮食及如何冲管
3. 掌握以下词汇

    obstructive jaundice　梗阻性黄疸
    endoscopic retrograde cholangiopancreatography (ERCP)　逆行性
       胰胆管造影
    nasal mucosa　鼻黏膜
    intact　完好无损的
    blood routine examination　血常规检查
    blood amylase　血淀粉酶

Li Ming is a patient with benign obstructive jaundice. On the second day after endoscopic retrograde cholangiopancreatography (ERCP) and endoscopic nasobiliary drainage (ENBD), Nurse Xiao Ran is providing nose and mouth care for him.

Xiao Ran: Li Ming, mouth care is done, and your nasal mucosa is intact. I just dripped compound mint oil to alleviate your nasal discomfort.

Li Ming: Thank you, Xiao Ran. For how many days will this tube stay in my body?

Xiao Ran: Usually three to five days. When your body temperature, blood routine examination results and blood amylase level are normal, there is no abdominal pain or bloating and the cholangiography results are normal, the tube will be removed.

Xiao Ran: Oh, you may eat some porridge today. Eat small but frequent meal. After eating, rinse your mouth to keep it clean.

Li Ming: Really? Is my blood amylase back to normal? Xiao Ran, may I ask you a question?

Xiao Ran: Of course.

Li Ming: If it gets blocked, do I have to undergo ERCP again?

Xiao Ran: Not always. Usually, we use a 20 mL syringe for low pressure suction. Then rinse with gentamicin in 0.9% sodium chloride solution at low pressure. If the drainage is not effective, we will consider replacing the tube.

李明是一位良性胆管梗阻性黄疸的患者，ERCP+ENBD 术后第 2 天，小冉护士正在为他做鼻腔和口腔护理。

小冉：李明，口腔护理已经做好，鼻腔黏膜完好，刚刚滴了复方薄荷油，以减轻鼻腔的不适感。

李明：谢谢你，小冉，这个管子要留几天啊？

小冉：一般 3～5 天。体温、血常规、血淀粉酶正常，无腹痛、腹胀，胆管造影结果正常就可以拔管了。

小冉：你今天可以喝点粥了，少食多餐，进食后及时漱口保持口腔清洁。

李明：真的吗？我的血淀粉酶恢复正常了？小冉，我可以问一个问题吗？

小冉：当然。

李明：如果阻塞，我是否需要再次接受 ERCP 手术？

小冉：不一定，通常我们会用 20 mL 注射器先低压抽取，再用 0.9% 生理盐水 + 庆大霉素低压冲洗，如果还是引流不畅，才会进一步考虑重新置管。

第三章　胃管

Chapter 3　Gastric tube

1. 熟悉胃管改良的方法
2. 鼻腔护理
3. 掌握以下词汇

intestinal obstruction　肠梗阻	aseptic procedures　无菌操作	
gastrointestinal decompression　胃肠减压	semi-reclining position　半卧位	
	menthol nasal　薄荷脑滴鼻剂	
nasal-gastric tube　鼻胃管		

Lu Xuan is a patient with advanced pancreatic cancer and has been taking painkillers for a long time. He has been diagnosed with intestinal obstruction. Gastrointestinal decompression is arranged using nasal-gastric tube. Lin Yun is his primary nurse. She is preparing for gastrointestinal decompression. She chooses 18 Fr gastric tube. Under aseptic procedures, two side holes are cut out from the blind side of the gastric tube and one side hole is expanded to ensure more effective drainage.

Nurse manager: Lin Yun, since the patient has a large body size, the placement of gastric tube should be 10 to 15 centimeters more than the distance of his nose-ear-subxiphoid. You need to put the patient in semi-reclining position when placing gastric tube.

Lin Yun: All right, nurse manager.

On the second day after gastrointestinal decompression, Lin Yun comes for a ward round.

Lu Xuan: Lin Yun, a nurse gave me oral care this morning. My mouth feels better now, but my nose still hurts.

Lin Yun: The doctor has prescribed menthol nasal drops to relieve dry pain in the nasal cavity. Now let me help you with nose drops.

Lu Xuan: Thanks. I hope it will make me feel better.

陆轩是一位胰腺癌晚期患者，长期服用止痛药，出现了肠梗阻，拟置入胃管进行胃肠减压。林允是他的责任护士，正在准备胃肠减压的用物，她选了 18 号胃管，在无菌操作下，为了引流更通畅，把胃管盲端剪了 2 个侧孔，扩大了 1 个侧孔。

护士长： 林允，这个患者体形高大，测量长度采用鼻－耳－剑突法，再加 10～15 cm，置入时，采取半卧位法。

林允： 好的，护士长。

胃肠减压第二天，林允去查房。

陆轩： 林允，早上有护士给我做了口腔护理，口腔清爽了很多，可我的鼻子不太舒服，有点疼。

林允： 医生给你开了薄荷脑滴鼻液，用来缓解鼻腔不适，现在我帮你滴一下鼻腔。

陆轩： 谢谢，希望它能让我好受点儿。

第四章 鼻空肠管

Chapter 4　Nasojejunal tube

📚 **学习目标** •

1. 掌握鼻空肠管常规护理
2. 熟悉堵管处理方法
3. 掌握以下词汇

enteral nutrition　肠内营养	adequately　充分的
syringe　注射器	rub　研磨
bowel peristalsis　肠蠕动	cram　填满
blockage　堵管	filtration　过滤

Liu Mei is a patient with acute pancreatitis. She will be returning home tomorrow with a nasojejunal tube for further nutritional therapy. Xiao Hui is a digestive specialist nurse. She will evaluate Liu Mei's management of nasojejunal tube today.

Xiao Hui: Now let's begin. Just relax.

Liu Mei: First, take out the nutrient solution from a cool and dry place. Nutrient solution should be prepared right before use. After removing the air from the infusion tube, pulse flush the tube using 20 mL warm drinking water with a 20 mL syringe. During the infusion process, repeat the flush every 4 hours. The temperature of nutrient solution should not be too high, between 37 to 40℃. Moderate exercises may be taken to promote bowel peristalsis during the infusion. Finally, flush the tube at the end of the infusion. Fix the tube with nasal patches. Record the exposed length of the tube, perinasal skin condition, infusion volume, and any discomfort such as abdominal pain on a daily basis.

Xiao Hui: Over time, tube blockage may occur. Two major causes of blockage are residue and incompletely crushed drug fragments adhering to the tube wall. The tablets should be thoroughly ground to prevent tube blockage caused by cramming of particles. Gauze filtration can be used if necessary. Well, Liu Mei, what should be done in case of blockage?

Liu Mei: Stop infusing and increase the frequency and volume of tube flushing until the blockage is gone.

Xiao Hui: Yes. If it is still blocked, you can inject 5% NaHCO$_3$ solution into the tube. Keep it sealed for 30 minutes and rinse with warm water. Or you can come to the hospital and ask us for help. Dial the number on the follow-up card in case you have any other problems.

Liu Mei: Thank you.

 译文

刘梅是一名急性胰腺炎患者，明天要带着鼻空肠管回家继续营养治疗。消化科护士小慧将评估刘梅营养管操作。

小慧： 现在开始吧，放松点。

刘梅： 首先，将营养液从阴凉干燥处取出，现用现配。排空输注管内的空气，输注前用 20 mL 注射器抽 20 mL 温开水脉冲式冲管，输注过程中每 4 小时冲管一次，输注温度为

37～40℃，温度不可过高，输注过程中可适当活动，促进肠蠕动。最后，输注结束后再次冲管，妥善固定鼻贴，每天记录管道的外露长度、鼻子周围的皮肤情况，输注量，有无腹痛等不适。

小慧： 时间久了，有可能会堵管，堵管的主要原因是残渣和粉碎不全的药物碎片黏附于管腔内，所以应充分研磨药片，避免颗粒导致堵管，必要时可用纱布过滤。那么刘梅，出现堵管时应如何处理？

刘梅： 应暂停输注，增加冲管的频率及量，直至管路通畅。

小慧： 是的，如果管路还是不通，可以推注 5% $NaHCO_3$ 溶液，封管保持 30 分钟，再用温水冲洗。你也可以直接来医院找我们，有其他任何问题都可以拨打随访卡上的电话咨询。

刘梅： 谢谢。

第五章 腹腔置管护理

Chapter 5 Abdominal catheter care

学习目标

1. 掌握腹腔置管的注意事项
2. 熟悉腹腔置管如何冲洗
3. 掌握以下词汇

debridement of peripancreatic necrosis 胰周坏死组织清除术

squeeze 挤压

hand hygiene 手部卫生

aseptic technique 无菌技术

Zhang Yi is a patient with severe acute pancreatitis complicated by abdominal infection. He underwent debridement of peripancreatic necrosis a week ago, and is currently in ICU. He has 3 drainage cannulas, which are right-side peripancreatic abscess cannula, right-side T-tube and right-side colon fistula cannula.

Li Li, an ICU nurse, is handing over work to the next shift with Liu Fen. She straightens out and fixes the drainage tubes on the abdominal wall with 3M tape using high platform method. The same drainage and inlet tubes are marked with the same color using color labels. The tube names and exposed lengths are also marked.

Liu Fen: Li Li, is there anything special about these drainage cannulas for shift handover?

Li Li: The smooth drainage of cannula must be ensured. Check drainage tubes once an hour. Squeeze drainage tubes constantly. Semi-recumbent position can be applied to facilitate drainage when vital signs are stable. Help the patient change positions per hour.

Liu Fen: How to flush the abdominal cannula?

Li Li: Dropping speed and negative pressure of flushing fluid should be adjusted timely according to the natures of the drainage fluid. The average speed is 25 to 50 drops per minute and the negative pressure is 10 to 20 kPa. The total amount of physiological saline per day is 2500 to 5000 mL.

Liu Fen: How to care for the skin around the catheter?

Li Li: Change dressings 1 to 2 times a day to keep them dry and clean. If necessary, apply zinc oxide to protect skin and prevent skin irritation caused by drainage fluid.

Liu Fen: Ok, I will keep that in mind.

Li Li: We must guarantee the hand hygiene of medical staff. Hand washing, or rapid hand disinfection is mandatory before and after operation or contact with patients. Aseptic technique should be properly employed.

张毅是一位重症急性胰腺炎合并腹腔感染的患者，1 周前行胰周坏死组织清除术，住在监护室，带有右胰周脓肿引流套管、右 T 管及右结肠瘘管。

李丽是 ICU 的护士，正在与刘芬交接班。她理顺并用 3M 胶布用高举平台法将引流管固定于腹壁上，采用彩色标识，同一根引流管和进水管贴同一颜色，标明管道名称及外露长度。

刘芬：李丽，这些管道有哪些特殊情况需要交班吗？

李丽：一定要确保导管引流通畅，每小时察看 1 次，经常挤压引流管，生命体征平稳后可取半坐卧位，每小时变换体位 1 次，以利于引流。

刘芬：平时如何冲洗呢？

李丽：冲洗液的滴速及负压根据引流液的性质随时做适当的调整，一般滴速为每分钟 25～50 滴，负压为 10～20 kPa，每天的生理盐水总量为 2 500～5 000 mL。

刘芬：置管处周围的皮肤如何护理呢？

李丽：每天换药 1～2 次，保持敷料干洁，必要时涂抹氧化锌保护皮肤，防止引流液腐蚀皮肤。

刘芬：好的，我会牢记在心。

李丽：要确保医护人员手卫生管理，操作前后、接触患者前后都要洗手或快速手消毒，严格无菌操作。

第六章 肝脓肿引流管

Chapter 6 Liver abscess drainage tube

1. 掌握肝脓肿的主要治疗
2. 熟悉留置肝脓肿引流管后的注意事项
3. 掌握以下词汇

liver/hepatic abscess　肝脓肿　　　fixator　固定器
antibiotic　抗生素

Tang Hua was diagnosed with liver abscess three days ago. He will undergo an operation for liver abscess tomorrow. His primary nurse Xu Juan is giving him a health instruction.

Tang Hua: Hi, Xu Juan. I have been using antibiotics for three days to avoid infection. What is the next treatment plan?

Xu Juan: Next, we need to puncture into the liver abscess and place a drainage tube for further treatment. We are planning to do it tomorrow.

Tang Hua: So soon? Then what do I need to do?

Xu Juan: Yes. I'm here just to tell you what to do. Avoid eating and drinking after tomorrow's operation. And a drainage tube for liver abscess will be attached to your abdomen when you come back. Since the tube is extremely important, we must prevent it from slipping. We will use a fixator to secure the tube to your abdominal skin. Then again, we use rubber bands and pins to fix the tube onto the bed sheet. You need to remove the pin when you turn over or get up to avoid pulling out the tube unexpectedly. We will pour the drainage liquid regularly. You can not turn on the switch of the tube by yourself.

Tang Hua: Thank you very much. I will bear your words in mind.

Xu Juan: You're welcome. Wish you a quick recovery.

唐华确诊肝脓肿 3 天了，明天就要做肝脓肿穿刺引流术。徐娟是他的责任护士，现在正在为唐华做健康宣教。

唐华： 你好，徐娟。我已经使用 3 天抗生素来控制炎症，接下来的治疗方案是什么？

徐娟： 接下来我们就要做肝脓肿穿刺并留置一根引流管，手术就在明天。

唐华： 这么快？那我需要做些什么呢？

徐娟： 是的，我就是来告诉你注意事项的。术后需要禁食、禁水，并且会带回一根肝脓肿引流管。这根引流管至关重要，我们一定要做好保护工作，避免滑脱。我们会使用固定器将导管固定在你腹部皮肤上，然后再用橡皮筋和别针将导管固定于床单上，进行双固定。你在翻身或者起床的时候需要将别针取下，以免脱出导管。我们也会及时倾倒引流液，你不可自行打开引流管上的开关。

唐华： 非常感谢你，我会牢记在心的。

徐娟： 不客气，祝你早日康复。

第七章 芒硝外敷护理

Chapter 7　Mirabilite topical care

1. 熟悉芒硝的作用机制
2. 掌握芒硝外敷的方法及注意事项
3. 掌握以下词汇

peritoneal effusion	腹部渗出	deliquesce	溶解
external application	外敷	osmotic pressure	渗透压
mirabilite	芒硝	inflammatory cytokines	炎性
osmosis	渗透作用		因子
freezing point	冰点	crystallize	结晶
absorbability	吸收性		

Su Fei is a patient with severe acute pancreatitis. She is conscious, but with huge abdominal bloating pain. CT scan shows massive peritoneal effusion. Li Mei is an ICU nurse. Bai Lu is a newly graduated intern.

Bai Lu: Ms. Li, what is mirabilite?

Li Mei: Well, mirabilite is a traditional Chinese medicine. Its chemical composition is Na_2SO_4 and other salts, colorless or white with strong osmosis and low freezing point. It has strong absorbability and is extremely easy to deliquesce. It can work for relieving constipation by purgation, moistening dryness, softening hardness, clearing fire, and reducing swelling.

Bai Lu: How does it absorb peritoneal effusion?

Li Mei: The osmotic pressure of mirabilite is significantly higher than that of human tissue. External application of mirabilite can create a local hypertonic environment. Osmotic pressure is applied to squeeze out tissue water, and promote the absorption of peritoneal effusion. What's more, external application of mirabilite can accelerate lymph circulation and improve the phagocytosis of reticuloendothelial cells, reduce the infiltration of white blood cells and promote the absorption of inflammatory cytokines.

Bai Lu: What about its usage and precautions?

Li Mei: Pack 1,000 g mirabilite into a cotton bag, then seal the bag before putting it evenly on the abdomen. Put a sanitary pad outside the cotton bag and cover it with the quilt. After 1 to 2 hours, when mirabilite is crystallized into crystal blocks or bag is wet, replace mirabilite and the bag. The total external application time is 8 to 10 hours per day.

Bai Lu: I see. Now I am going to get mirabilite ready for Su Fei.

苏菲是一个重症急性胰腺炎的患者，神志清，但是腹部剧烈胀痛，CT 提示腹腔积液较多。李梅是一名 ICU 的护士，白露是一名刚毕业的实习生。

白露：李老师，芒硝是什么？

李梅：芒硝是一味中药，它的化学成分主要是 Na_2SO_4 等盐类，无色或白色，渗透性强，冰点低，吸收性好，极易潮解。有泻下通便、润燥软坚、清火消肿的功能。

白露：它是怎么吸收腹腔积液呢？

李梅：芒硝的晶体渗透压显著高于人体组织渗透压，芒硝外敷可以在局部形成高渗环境，借助渗透压的作用使组织水分渗出体外，从而促使腹腔积液吸收。而且，芒硝外敷时能加快淋巴循环，提高网状内皮细胞的吞噬功能，减少白细胞浸润，促进炎性细胞因子的吸收。

白露：它的使用方法和注意事项呢？

李梅：芒硝 1 000 g，均匀装入棉布袋中，封闭后平铺于腹部，布袋外面放置卫生垫，盖好被子，外敷 1～2 小时芒硝凝结成结晶块，或棉布袋潮湿，要更换芒硝及布袋，每天外敷总时间 8～10 小时。

白露：明白了，我这就去给苏菲准备芒硝等物品。

第八章　PTCD 管

Chapter 8　Percutaneous transhepatic cholangial drainage tube (PTCD tube)

1. 熟悉 PTCD 作用
2. 掌握 PTCD 置管期间体位与活动
3. 掌握饮食指导
4. 了解导管的护理
5. 掌握以下词汇

X-ray fluoroscopy	X 线引导下	supine position	仰卧位
B-ultrasound guidance	B 超引导下	diarrhea	腹泻

Li Ming suffers from malignant obstructive jaundice and has undergone percutaneous transhepatic cholangial drainage (PTCD). Xiao Ran is his primary nurse. PTCD is a technique for percutaneous transhepatic puncture of bile ducts and placement of drainage tubes under the guidance of imaging equipment (usually X-ray fluoroscopy or B-ultrasound guidance) to drain bile out of the body or into duodenum. The patient's jaundice is obviously alleviated. Abdominal bloating is relieved and liver function is improved. He has increased appetite and improved mood.

Xiao Ran: Hi Li Ming, how are you feeling now?

Li Ming: Not too bad. But I do not dare to move.

Xiao Ran: Take it easy. Maintain supine position in the initial 6 hours after surgery. The drainage bag should be lower than the puncture site when you get out of bed, and it should be lower than the midaxillary line when you lie down.

Li Ming: Thank you. Can I drink water now?

Xiao Ran: You should fast in the first 8 hours after operation. Then choose low fat diet with sufficient calorie, protein, and vitamin. Eat small but frequent meals of digestible food. You may gradually transition to regular diet if there is no abdominal bloating, diarrhea, or other discomfort. Be sure to avoid high fat diet.

Li Ming: Is there anything else I should pay attention to?

Xiao Ran: First, the catheter should be fixed properly and kept unblocked. Reversal and distortion should be avoided. Second, observe the color, nature and quantity of the drainage liquid. Finally, seek help from your doctor whenever you do not feel good.

Li Ming: Thank you very much.

　　李明患有恶性梗阻性黄疸、已接受了经皮肝穿刺胆道引流术（PTCD），小冉是他的责任护士。PTCD 是在影像设备（通常为 X 线透视下或 B 超引导下）引导下经皮经肝穿刺胆管并置入引流管，使胆汁流向体外或十二指肠的技术。患者黄疸明显减退，腹胀缓解，肝功能改善，食欲提高，心情也好多了。

小冉：你好，李明，现在感觉怎么样？

李明：还好，我现在不敢活动。

小冉：别紧张，术后 6 小时保持平卧，如果要下床活动，引流袋要低于穿刺部位，平卧时要低于腋中线。

李明：谢谢，我现在能喝水吗？

小冉：术后 8 小时禁食、禁水，饮食以低脂、高热量、高蛋白质、高维生素、易消化、少食多餐为原则，如无腹胀、腹泻等不适主诉，逐渐过渡到普食，忌高脂饮食。

李明：我还有其他需要注意的吗？

小冉：首先，导管要固定好，保持通畅，避免反折、扭曲；其次，观察引流液的颜色、性质和量；最后，如果有其他不适症状，及时告知医生。

李明：非常感谢！

第九章　小肠减压管
Chapter 9　Small intestinal decompression tube

 学习目标

1. 了解小肠减压管的结构及作用
2. 掌握腹痛、腹胀症状的原因
3. 熟悉小肠减压管的留置时间
4. 掌握以下词汇

stomach pylorus　胃幽门	bowel sounds　肠鸣音
alleviate　减轻	paraffin oil　石蜡油

Li Ming is a patient with small intestinal obstruction and has undergone intestinal decompression tube replacement. Xiao Ran is his primary nurse. The 3-meter long small intestinal decompression tube consists of two sacs and three cavities with a 3.5 m guide wire. The front end is a bead shaped guide with a stainless-steel ball, which can pass through the stomach pylorus and move under the force of intestinal peristalsis. The nasal-small intestine decompression tube will enter the small intestine through the pylorus. The drainage of intestinal content can decrease the pressure in the gastrointestinal cavity, improve the local blood circulation, and alleviate the symptoms of intestinal obstruction.

Xiao Ran: Hi, Li Ming. The imaging shows that the small

intestinal decompression tube has reached the obstruction position, and has been secured.

Li Ming: Thank you, Xiao Ran. My abdomen is still bloated and distended. I am wondering when the symptoms will be relieved.

Xiao Ran: It may take 48 to 72 hours.

Li Ming: Oh, I see. And when will the tube be pulled out?

Xiao Ran: It depends on how well you recover. The signs of recovery include alleviated abdominal bloating and pain, voluntary defecation and exhaust, normalized bowel sounds, disappearance of gas-liquid level under X-ray observation. You need to drink 100 to 150 mL of paraffin oil 1 to 2 hours before extubating. We will extract distilled water from the anterior balloon and apply intermittent extubation to avoid possible discomfort.

Li Ming: Ok, I hope this moment will come soon.

Xiao Ran: Yes, we are all looking forward to it.

Li Ming: Thank you.

　　李明是一位小肠梗阻患者，小肠减压管术后，小冉是他的责任护士。全长 3 cm 的小肠减压管包含两囊三腔，配有长度为 3.5 m 的导丝，前端为念珠状前导子，含不锈钢球，可通过胃部幽门并在肠蠕动的推动力下运动，引流管处接胃肠减压器。鼻小肠减压管经幽门进入小肠。肠道内容物引流可降低胃肠腔内压力，改善局部血液循环，解除肠梗阻症状。

　　小冉：李明，影像片提示小肠减压管已到梗阻位置，管道也固定得很好。

李明：谢谢小冉。我现在腹部还是很胀，我想知道这种症状何时缓解？

小冉：可能需要 48～72 小时。

李明：哦，我知道了，这个管子什么时候能拔掉？

小冉：根据你恢复的情况来定。比如说腹部胀痛症状缓解、自主排便排气、肠鸣音正常、X 线提示气液平面消失。拔管前 1～2 小时内需要口服石蜡油 100～150 mL。我们会抽出前球囊内的蒸馏水，采用间歇性拔管方式，避免出现不适症状。

李明：好的，我希望这个时刻早点到来。

小冉：是的，我们都很期待。

李明：谢谢。